THE

By-Your-Side

CANCER
GUIDE

THE

By-Your-Side

CANCER GUIDE

Empowered, Proactive, Prepared

Deborah Gomer, BSN, RN, OCN, CCM, CHC

Cunningham House Publishing
St. Johns, Florida

Published by:
Cunningham House Publishing
www.deborahgomer.com

Printed in the United States of America
First Printing, 2018

Paperback ISBN: 978-0-9995998-0-8
eBook ISBN: 978-0-9995998-1-5

Library of Congress Cataloging-in-Publication Data has been applied for.

Cover Design: Kerrianne Bowen
Interior Design: Ghislain Viau

To Howard, Amanda, Jerry, and Dad.

Your love, encouragement, laughter,
and support bring light and joy into my life.

Thank you for believing in me.

Contents

Part I: Getting Started

Part II: Caring for Your Mind

Part III: Caring for Your Body

Part IV: Addressing Difficult Issues

Part V: Life Beyond Cancer

Foreword

When you get a cancer diagnosis, it is most likely one of the scariest times of your life. It has been so comforting to have someone outside of my family who is completely objective but so incredibly compassionate and understanding about what I have been going through as an individual. She helped me to stay focused and take one step at a time. Years of experience as an oncology nurse have given Debbie a real understanding of what her patients deal with on a regular basis. She is full of sound advice on how to handle many different problems and side effects that come from treatment and medication, as well as the emotional trauma that comes with such a diagnosis. Debbie has been a godsend to me and I am so thankful she has written this book. There is no doubt this will be such a help to so many.

Paula Marion, breast cancer survivor

Preface

I graduated from New York University with a Bachelor of Science in Nursing degree in 1988. Right away, I knew what I was going to do—specialize in oncology. Oncology encompassed everything that was wonderful about being a nurse. It was challenging, requiring keen assessment skills, the ability to teach with patience, the willingness to continue learning, and a lot of compassion. It was a choice that seemed to fit me well. Since graduation, I have worked in almost every subspecialty of oncology—chemotherapy, education, research, transplant, home health, hospice, and case management. This is truly what I was meant to do.

In 2006, I found myself in a new role. I was no longer just an oncology nurse, I was the oncology patient. You see, I have a condition called dysplastic nevus syndrome, also known as atypical mole syndrome. Lucky me. Most people have a few moles on their body. People with dysplastic nevus syndrome have hundreds of moles.

These moles can vary in size and color and are often abnormal. According to the National Organization for Rare Disorders, individuals with this syndrome have a higher risk of developing melanoma.

I had been seeing a dermatologist every six months since I was in my twenties. For me, it was just routine for moles to be removed and biopsied, and usually they were dysplastic, abnormal. Once removed, they were gone and forgotten. But this one day in April, as I was heading home with my young son from an appointment, I got the dreaded call: One of my moles turned out to be malignant melanoma. My first feeling was numbness, as if I were in a dream. What would I do when I got home? How would I tell my husband? My thought were racing.

Ironically, the diagnosis came just after my family decided to join the local American Cancer Society Race for the Cure. How strange it felt to be diagnosed with cancer and walking the track before I had told anyone. Besides, I'm an oncology nurse. We nurses take care of others. We don't play patient very well. I was used to being in the driver's seat, but I was being pushed into the passenger's seat. Part of me wanted to take charge and another part wanted someone to take my hand a lead the way. I realized I had to be in the driver's seat to get through it. But I needed a plan.

Did I cry? Sure I did. Cancer really does suck. Being an oncology nurse with cancer really, really sucks. We know way too much for our own good. We typically see patients who have advanced disease. So, of course, I prepared myself for the worst. But I also refused to let this cancer thing either define or get the best of me.

If I was going to get through this, I was going to need to do it with knowledge, strength, and humor. I was going to be empowered, proactive, and prepared.

I did as much research as I could. I asked questions. I accepted love and support from family and friends. I pretty much held it together, except when I did the what-ifs. What if it was advanced? What if I am disfigured? What about my kids? My husband?

I decided up front that I was going to shut out those who had only negative comments. And there were plenty of negative, or should I say ignorant, comments. I had been teaching Zumba at the time of my diagnosis. After confiding in one of my clients, she responded with, "Oh, my sister had melanoma. It went to her brain and she died." Hmm, that was helpful to hear. I was also taking martial arts classes at the time. My classmates ignored the subject. No one asked how I was doing. No one called when I missed class. And no one asked how I was when I returned. Even one of my family members commented, "It's not like you are dying or anything." It was as if by ignoring my situation, these people did not have to face their own mortality.

At the same time, there were people who rallied around me and my family. Without being asked, neighbors would take my son for a few hours so I could rest. And some family members and friends would call on a regular basis just to check in.

My surgery took place in June of 2006. My mole was smaller than a pencil eraser, but because melanoma is a sneaky bugger, it is important to remove a fairly good amount of surrounding tissue.

Because my mole was close to my neck, I was placed under the care of a head and neck surgeon. My incision extended along the jaw line and I had several lymph nodes removed. My face was swollen, bruised, and disfigured after surgery. It took a while to be able to regain full range of motion of my neck or be able to swallow without discomfort. But I think the absolute worst part was waiting for the results of the lymph node biopsies. If they were positive, I had some serious thinking to do because treatment for malignant melanoma was limited and not very effective at the time.

One week later I found myself shaking in the surgeon's office. He looked at me, smiled, and calmly told me that my lymph node biopsies were negative and the area surrounding the malignant mole was clear. He gave me a big hug and told me to go home and get on with my life. *Oh my gosh!* My heart started to beat again. I was actually breathing. But anyone who has had cancer knows you never truly put this entire saga behind you.

I am now at an even greater risk of developing another melanoma and will always be at risk of the original melanoma showing up in another organ. As much as I try, I will always hold thoughts in the back of my head that an ache or a pain could mean more than it really does. I continue to see the dermatologist several times a year, and nothing is taken lightly. In fact, the dermatology surgeon did not want to take any chances and opted to remove two more very large moles just after I healed from the melanoma surgery. One was on my buttock and the other on my pelvic area. Let me tell you, it was miserable. I had to resort to wearing nothing but sweat pants for 2 months because I could not have anything touch the incisions.

Walking was difficult too. As of today, I have had over 50 biopsies and have over 50 scars to prove it. At times I feel self-conscious. At times I curse the scars and this stupid disease. But I never stop feeling blessed because, despite those scars, I am here. Life is truly a gift and there is so much joy to be had in each day.

So I can truly say that cancer sucks. I know it because I have lived with it—the anxiety, uncertainty, physical scars, and emotional pain. I also know this because I am an oncology nurse and a case manager. I have learned a lot from my patients and my fellow nurses. I have also gained a new perspective on the cancer experience. I have listened to my patients and identified the questions and concerns that have been most pressing. I have received input as to what information has helped them the most.

In writing this book, I am sharing what I have learned from my patients and from my personal experience. I have included tips and suggestions that will help you manage your diagnosis and care for your mind and body. I hope this book informs and inspires you to become empowered, proactive, and prepared.

Introduction

When you live with cancer, life becomes a series of questions. How do I understand my insurance? How do I choose a physician? What is the best treatment plan? How do I manage symptoms and side effects?

Then there are the questions that tend to be avoided. How do I deal with my feelings? How do I keep my spirits up? How do I address intimacy and sexuality? What if my cancer recurs?

Volumes of books address cancer. Some are written by celebrities, some by physicians or nurses, and others by patients. There are books that advise what to eat and what not to eat. There are books that discuss specific cancers. There are books that provide emotional support. So why another cancer book?

As an oncology nurse and cancer survivor, I have been on both sides of the spectrum. I understand the fear and uncertainty. In my search for a resource to recommend to my patients, I have been unable to find a book that answers all of the questions my patients had been asking me. So I set out to chart a comprehensive course for coping with a cancer diagnosis. Within these pages, you will find information on the first steps to take after diagnosis. You will find information on insurance, choosing a treatment plan, managing side effects, and nourishing your body. You will also find information on sexuality, advanced cancer, and ways to care for your spirit. The appendix section includes a list of resources, a glossary, and some simple recipes to help you along the way. This book is not meant to be read from cover to cover, but used as a resource to refer to throughout your cancer journey. Pick and choose the chapters that resonate with you.

My intention is for this book to serve as a compassionate, concise guide to strengthen your mind, body, and spirit so you can be empowered to take control of your medical care and your life. Many patients face a similar question: Where do I start? Having a plan is of the utmost importance. By knowing where to begin and how to be proactive, you will be prepared to be your own best advocate from those critical first steps. Let this be the guide you keep by your side from the start to help navigate your way through your cancer journey. Let's get started.

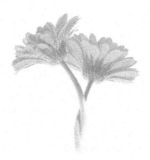

Part I

Getting Started

Chapter 1

The First Steps

By knowing where to begin, and how to be proactive, you will be prepared to be your own best advocate. The first steps in your cancer journey will help empower you to take charge of your medical care:

1. Choose your cancer buddy.
2. Put together your treatment team.
3. Contact your insurance company and learn about your benefits.
4. Ask questions.
5. Stay organized.
6. Nurture your mind and body.

This may seem daunting, but you can and must take charge of your health from the beginning. Let's explore each of these in greater detail.

Step 1—Choose Your Cancer Buddy

The first step in your cancer journey will be to choose a cancer buddy. A buddy can be a spouse, significant other, sibling, friend, parent, family member, or anyone who can join hands with you along this journey. Let your buddy know what you will need to help you through the decision making process. Have them accompany you during initial appointments and consultations.

If you do not have someone available to be your buddy, you do not need to go it alone. Find out if your insurance company offers nurse case management as part of your benefit plan. If so, take advantage of this cost-free service. I have worked as a nurse case manager for 15 years and find this to be one of the most rewarding jobs I have ever had. Nurse case managers can provide telephonic support, walking you through each step of your journey. They can provide education and resources for you to become your best advocate. Nurse case managers can also help advocate on your behalf. They can even help you understand your insurance benefits. Even if you have a cancer buddy, you might still consider enrolling in a nurse case management program because nurse case managers can provide support to you and your buddy.

Nurse navigators or patient navigators are another option to help you as you start your cancer journey. Many cancer treatment centers offer the services of a navigator to guide people through the first steps of their cancer journey. They may help set up initial appointments and coordinate care with insurance companies. They may explain your diagnosis and treatment options and help you understand what you can expect. Some navigators function as social workers, providing information about community resources and financial assistance. Many cancer centers employ navigators, so ask if one is available to you.

So now you have your buddy. What's next?

Step 2—Put Together Your Treatment Team

Once you have been diagnosed, your physician will recommend a next step. Quite often, the next step may be a referral to a surgeon. If you have not been referred to a medical oncologist, you should include one as part of your treatment team. Surgeons are experts at surgery. Radiation oncologists are experts at radiation treatment. Medical oncologists see the overall picture. A medical oncologist can give you a better understanding of your diagnosis, treatment options, and prognosis. A medical oncologist will also oversee the coordination of your care, referring you to specialists, as needed, and will continue to follow up with you after treatment is complete.

You can, and should, contact your insurance company for a list of in-network providers. Ask your primary care physician or treating physician for a recommendation. If you know someone who has been treated for cancer, get their input on where to seek treatment. Your oncology team will be an important part of your cancer journey and feeling comfortable with the doctors and the staff is important. Most insurance companies allow for a second or even a third opinion. Take advantage of this and consider consulting two or three doctors before you make your decision.

Cancer care can be rendered in a variety of settings. Some physicians are in group practice, working with several physicians in the same specialty of practice. Some are part of a comprehensive cancer center where the focus is providing a full spectrum of cancer care. Comprehensive cancer centers may include medical oncologists, radiation oncologists, lab technicians, social workers, and nurse navigators under one roof. Other oncologists practice in an academic setting where they are part of a university center.

When choosing your oncologist and cancer treatment center, consider how far you are willing to travel for your care. You may consider traveling to a major cancer center for a consultation, especially if you have advanced cancer or a rare type of cancer. It is possible to see an oncologist at a major cancer center for your treatment plan, then have the actual treatment administered locally. If you will be receiving radiation therapy or chemotherapy, you may not want to drive several hours for your care. Traveling great distances for care is not always necessary. A doctor's bedside manner may be just as important as the place in which he or she practices.

This is your first opportunity to take charge of your medical care. Commit to being an active participant. Most people feel health care decisions are the responsibility of their medical team. Ultimately, you are responsible for your health and the decisions surrounding it. Choose a medical team who you trust and who welcomes your questions and responds to your concerns.

Step 3—Contact Your Insurance Company and Learn About Your Benefits

No matter what type of facility you choose, contact your insurance company and make sure both the physician and the facility are in-network. You will also want to make sure the diagnostic centers and labs you use are in-network. Some insurance plans have out-of-network benefits, but significant differences in the coverage could leave you with a larger out-of-pocket expense. You will also want to find out about co-pays and deductibles. If this sounds foreign to you, the next chapter will explain insurance and benefits in depth.

Step 4—Ask Questions

Cancer treatment is individualized and based on specific criteria, including the cancer site, cell type, stage of disease, age, other medical conditions, and any previous treatment. You may know someone who had the same type of cancer as you, but their treatment plan may not be the same as yours. Talking with others who have had your type of cancer can be helpful and supportive, but each person's treatment and experience will be different. By educating yourself about your diagnosis, you can become an active participant in making treatment decisions. This is your life and your body. No matter how overwhelming your diagnosis may feel, you can maintain control by empowering yourself with the knowledge you need to make decisions about your care.

Bring a notebook and your list of questions to your first appointment. If possible, bring your cancer support buddy. Four ears are better than two. Knowledge truly is power. Stay informed about your cancer type and the treatment options that are available. The following is a list of questions you may want to ask during your initial appointments with your oncology team. We will address these questions in more depth in the following chapters:

- What type of cancer do I have? What organs are involved?
- What is the stage of my cancer?

- What is the goal of treatment?
- What treatment options are available for my stage of cancer?
- How often will the treatment be given?
- What side effects should I expect and how will it impact my daily life?
- What is my prognosis?
- How will you monitor my progress and what tests will be ordered?
- What type of support is available to me and my family?
- Who do I talk with in regards to insurance, billing, and financial assistance?

The internet is full of information, but the amount can be overwhelming. You may also get input from friends, family, and acquaintances. It is easy to get overburdened with information, especially when information is negative or conflicting. How do you digest all of this information? Stay educated and informed, but allow your oncology team to guide you through your cancer journey so that you make the best decisions for you. The American Cancer Society, National Cancer Institute, and National Comprehensive Cancer Network are reputable sources that provide educational material about cancer types and treatment options. You can find their websites listed under Appendix C: Resources in the back of this book.

Step 5—Stay Organized

Keep all of your medical records in one place. It could be a binder, a folder, your computer or tablet. Some hospitals and cancer centers give their patients access to a patient portal which allows patients to manage their medical records online. The portal may give other physicians in the hospital system a way to stay updated on your care, and it gives you a way of viewing physician notes, diagnostic tests, and labs. If you have access to a patient portal, you would still need a system to organize bills, insurance information, and any other papers pertaining to your care. Whatever system you choose, make sure that you keep your medical information updated.

Here is a sample list of some items you may want to keep in your folder or binder:

- Contacts and resources
- Business cards for each member of your cancer care team
- Insurance information and contact numbers
- Calendar to keep track of appointments
- Treatment information, including dates, type of treatment, the physician, and names of drugs/chemotherapy
- Medical history—Ask your oncologist for a copy of the consultation note.
- Test results and pathology reports—Ask your physician for copies of reports.
- CD holder to store copies of scans
- Medication list—You may choose to keep a written or typed list of medications in a folder. Do make sure to update the list with each medication change. Consider taking a picture of the list and keep it stored on your smartphone.

Step 6—Nurture Your Mind and Body

Commit to being an active participant in your care. Most people feel their health care decisions are the responsibility of their medical team. Remember, you are responsible for your health and decisions surrounding it. Your medical team will be a vital part of your treatment, but your decisions and actions will play a core part in achieving wellness.

Adopt a holistic principle of caring for yourself. That means caring for your mind and your body. It means integrating complementary therapies into your treatment plan to boost your immune system and optimize your overall health. Conventional treatment addresses your disease. Complementary treatment addresses you, the person. Emotions, relationships, and beliefs play a big role in how you heal. Having a cancer diagnosis feels like you have lost control, and caring for your mind and body gives you back that sense of control.

Chapter 2

Managing the Cost of Care

Right now, you need to focus on wellness and prioritize your health. That may be easier said than done when you are concerned about bills, expenses, and employment. Let's face it—it's hard to concentrate on getting well when you are worried about how you are going to pay for your care and your living expenses. Case managers talk to their patients every day about insurance, resources, and employment issues because these worries can be as real and as big as the cancer itself. So, before we move forward, we need to address insurance and financial issues.

First things first: Call your insurance company and ask to be assigned a case manager. The case manager can help you make sense of benefits and give you guidance in navigating the health care system. If your cancer treatment center has a nurse navigator or social worker, set up an appointment. This will give you the opportunity to learn about resources that may be available through the treatment center and the community. Case managers, nurse navigators, and social workers can be your advocates in obtaining services and care.

The next step is to learn how to access your benefit information, too. Does your insurance company have a website? Get familiar with the information on the website. Most insurance websites allow you to search for in-network physicians and facilities, check your claims, and learn about your benefits. If you are not comfortable on a computer, you can call member benefits or member services for assistance. The number can be found on your insurance card. A piece of advice here—always write down the name of the person you spoke with, the date, and the information given. Keep this in a file for easy access. (Remember we talked about the importance of staying organized?)

Insurance companies commonly revise their benefit offerings, coverage, and premiums from year to year. Be aware of any changes so you are not caught off-guard.

Important to note is that health care coverage in the United States is in a state of change. At the time of this writing, the below information was the most current information available. You are encouraged to visit the websites listed throughout this chapter for the most up-to-date information.

Understanding Insurance Terminology

Do you have a PPO? HMO? Fee-for-service plan?

PPO stands for Preferred Physician Organization. This plan allows you the freedom to choose your physicians from a list of network physicians. Some PPO's allow you to seek care out-of-network, but you will be responsible for a larger dollar amount. Each plan differs, so it is important to know whether you have out-of-network benefits. You do not need a referral to see a physician with this type of plan.

HMO stands for Health Maintenance Organization. Care under an HMO plan is covered only if you see an in-network physician. There are no out-of-network benefits. Most HMO plans require that you choose a primary care physician (PCP) and obtain a written referral before seeing a specialist.

Fee-for-service plans require the patient to pay for services out-of-pocket and the insurance company will provide reimbursement. The cost of care is based on a negotiated rate with the insurance company.

What is a premium? Deductible? Co-pay?

A premium is the amount you pay each month for your insurance coverage. And a deductible is the amount you will be expected to pay out-of-pocket before your insurance begins to pay. The amount varies depending on your plan. Contact your insurance company to find out the amount of your deductible.

Once you have met your deductible, you will be responsible for a co-payment, or co-pay. Although your insurance company will cover the majority of your health care costs, you will still be responsible for a portion. It may be a fixed amount (for example, $40 for each visit to a medical specialist), or it may be a percentage (for example, 20% for diagnostic tests).

What Are Your Options If You Can No Longer Work?

If you are not able to continue working, you may have options to consider.

Family Medical Leave Act (FMLA) entitles eligible employees to take unpaid time off for specific family-related or medical-related reasons. If you qualify, you may take up to 12 weeks of unpaid leave in a 12-month period. This leave cannot be counted against you. Your original job, or an equivalent job, must be provided to you upon your return. You may be required to use up vacation time or paid-time-off (PTO) before you can use FMLA.

In order to qualify for FMLA, the following criteria must be met:

- You must work for an employer who has at least 50 employees working within a 75 mile radius.
- You must have worked for this employer for at least 12 months prior to requesting FMLA.
- You must have worked an average of 24 hours per week in a 12-month period.
- You can find more information at the U.S. Department of Labor website, www.dol.gov. Contact your Human Resources department to find out if you are eligible.

Consolidated Omnibus Reconciliation Act (COBRA) allows you to keep your current medical insurance and benefits should you lose your job or need to leave your job. Sounds great, right? But this is what you need to know: You should be eligible if you work for an employer who has at least 20 employees. In order to keep your current insurance plan, with all of the same benefits, you must pay the entire premium—your cost plus the amount your employer had been paying. It is expensive, but it does allow you to continue coverage for 18 months if your employment ends or your hours are reduced.

Following are important points to note:

- You have an election period (usually 60 days) in which you can decide whether to elect COBRA. Use this time to look at all of your options. You may be eligible for private insurance, Medicare, or Medicaid. You can also look at the health insurance marketplace to find and compare insurance options through the Affordable Care Act (ACA) health exchanges. Visit www.healthcare.gov or call 1-800-318-2596 for more information about the Marketplace.

- Under the Health Insurance Portability Act (HIPPA), you cannot be denied coverage for a pre-existing condition. But keep in mind that you must have had medical coverage for at least 12 months and cannot have a lapse in coverage that exceeds 63 days.

- *Short-term Disability (STD) and Long-term Disability (LTD)*: Short-term disability is a type of insurance benefit that pays a percentage of employee salaries if they are unable to work due to illness or injury. Some employers require that vacation days and accrued sick days be used before short-term disability begins. This benefit may pay 40-60% of the employee's salary. The length of coverage may vary from 9 to 52 weeks, depending on the employer's policy. Long-term disability would kick in once the short-term coverage expires. Like short-term disability, it covers a percentage of the employee's salary for a designated period of time. Employers are not required to offer short- or long-term disability. Check with your employer's human resources department to find out if you are eligible, how you apply, and what your benefits include.

Are You Eligible For Medicare?

Medicare is a federally funded program that is available to those who meet the following criteria:

- You qualify for Medicare benefits at age 65 if you are a U.S. citizen and have lived in the U.S. for at least five years, and you or your spouse has worked long enough to qualify for Social Security benefits—about 10 years.

- You qualify for Medicare benefits under age 65 if you have received Social Security Disability (SSDI) benefits for 24 months, you receive disability from the Railroad Retirement Board, or you have Lou Gehrig's disease or end stage renal disease requiring dialysis.

What Are The Different Parts of Medicare?

Part A: Medicare Part A covers hospital care, hospice, home health care, and in-patient rehabilitation and skilled nursing care at a Medicare-accredited facility. There is no monthly premium, but you must meet an annual deductible.

Part B: Medicare Part B covers doctor visits, out-patient services, out-patient rehabilitation therapy, diagnostic tests, physician services, medical equipment, ambulance services and specialty medications—like chemotherapy. Part B coverage is optional and the premium is based on your income.

Part C: Medicare Part C is also known as Medicare Advantage. It is a Medicare program managed by Medicare-approved companies. It provides Medicare Parts A and B, as well as Medicare Part D, which is prescription coverage. There is a monthly premium based on the type of Medicare plan. Plans may be PPO, HMO, or fee-for-services. Some plans may even include coverage for vision, dental, and/or hearing.

Part D: Medicare Part D is prescription coverage. There is a monthly premium based on income, an annual deductible, and possibly a co-pay for drugs.

Where Can You Go To Find Out More About Medicare?

The government website www.medicare.gov provides more information. If you prefer to have your questions answered through a live chat, you can visit www.mymedicare.gov. You can also call 1-800-MEDICARE (1-800-633-4227). The National Council on Aging provides a wealth of information on their Medicare Matters website at www.mymedicarematters.org.

What Is Medicaid?

This government funded program provides coverage for low-income families, Supplemental Security Income (SSI) recipients, and certain individuals who fall under the poverty level. To see if you qualify, call 1-800-318-2596 or visit The Healthcare Market-place at www.healthcare.gov.

What Is SSI?

SSI stands for Supplemental Security Income and is not the same as SSDI. It is a federal program that provides monthly cash assistance to people who are disabled, blind, or elderly and have a very limited income and very little assets. If your disability prevents you from performing any type of gainful work and you can demonstrate financial need, you may want to consider applying for SSI. You can call 1-800-772-1213 or visit www.ssa.gov.

What Is SSDI?

This is Social Security Disability Income. It provides monthly payments to people who meet certain criteria for disability and are no longer able to work. If you have worked for any length of time, you may be eligible for SSDI.

Although cancer can be debilitating, and it may interfere with your ability to continue working during treatment, it does not guarantee that you will qualify for disability benefits through Social Security.

The following criteria must be met in order to qualify for SSDI:
- The cancer must be inoperable, recurrent, or have distant spread (metastases).
- The applicant must also show that he/she is not doing substantial work at the time of the application.
- There are some medical conditions and specific types of cancer that would automatically qualify an applicant for approval.

If you have advanced cancer, you may be eligible for expedited benefits through the Compassionate Allowances program. If you qualify, you would receive a response to your application in as little as 10 days. Keep in mind that your physician must supply your medical records. If there is a delay in sending information, it could also delay a response from Social Security. Once Social Security issues an approval, you must wait at least five months from the disability date to receive your benefits. Medicare benefits kick in 24 months after the disability date, so you would need insurance coverage to fill in the gap.

3 ways to apply for SSDI:

1. Visit the local Social Security office. You may be able to avoid a long wait by calling ahead to schedule an appointment.
2. Apply online at www.ssa.gov. The website offers a lot of information to help you decide if SSDI is right for you.
3. Call 1-800-772-1213, and ask for a phone appointment to speak with a Social Security case worker who can help you with the application. This also gives you a point of contact.

Financial Assistance

Even with insurance, the cost of medical care can be devastating. If you find that you need financial assistance, ask your physician to refer you to a social worker or a navigator. If you are admitted to a hospital, call the hospital billing department to find out if you qualify for financial assistance. Many hospitals and treatment facilities will work out a payment plan based on what you can afford to pay each month. Many drug companies offer patient assistance programs to help defray the costs of their medications. These programs require an application and you must show financial need.

Plan to spend some time searching for resources. Many organizations provide assistance for specific cancer diagnoses. The American Cancer Society (1-800-227-2345 or www.cancer.org) can provide information as to what resources may be available in your area. Cancer Care (1-800-813-4673 or www.cancercare.org) offers access to a social worker for free. Call your utility companies and explain that you are undergoing treatment for cancer. You may qualify for assistance. The website www.cancerfac.org is a coalition of organizations helping cancer patients manage their financial challenges. The Patient Advocate Foundation (1-800-532-5274 or www.patientadvocate.org) offers the ability to chat with case managers who specialize in helping with insurance-related issues and questions. The website also houses a financial resource directory.

Understanding Authorizations
And Appeals

Diagnostic tests, medical procedures, and treatments may require prior authorization from your insurance company. The ordering physician's responsibility is to obtain authorizations from your insurance company prior to rendering treatment or performing procedures or surgery. To avoid aggravation and frustration, call your physician's office prior to your scheduled treatment, procedure, or admission to make sure the authorization has been obtained. It's also a good idea to make sure the facility and physician are in-network. A nurse case manager can be instrumental assisting in this process. If at this point you have not already done so, contact your insurance company to see if a case manager is available to you.

If your insurance company denies an authorization, contact your physician's office and request that they initiate an appeal. The physician may also request a peer-to-peer review. This gives the physician the opportunity to speak with the insurance company's medical director, one-on-one, and discuss your case. Inform your nurse case manager, if you are working with one, in order to get further guidance in managing the denial.

Medication Challenges

Some medications require prior authorization. Medications, such as narcotic pain medications, have a limit on how many pills can be dispensed at a time and how often you can obtain a refill. To avoid unnecessary hassles, follow these tips:

- Ask your physician if any of the prescriptions you have been given require prior authorization. Your pharmacist can also inform you of any prior authorization requirements. The ordering physician's office must contact the insurance company to initiate any required prior authorization request. Once the authorization is processed, you should be able to obtain your prescription.

- If your insurance company limits the amount of pills you can obtain, or has limited the frequency of refills, ask your physician's office to call the insurance company and request an override, which will allow you to obtain the entire prescription amount.

- If your insurance company denies a medication, inform your physician, as there may be an equally effective alternative that would be covered. If you must have that specific medication, your physician's office can call the insurance company and explain why the medication is medically necessary.

Resources That May Help Defray The Cost Of Medications

If you are not able to afford a particular medication, ask for the assistance of a social worker, navigator, or case manager who may be able to provide resources to help defray the cost. Many pharmaceutical companies have patient assistance programs. You can find information by typing the name of the medication, followed by "patient assistance" in your computer's search engine. You can also ask your pharmacist to help find a contact number for you. You will find more resources in the Appendix C: Resource section of this book.

Chapter 3

Understanding
Your Treatment Options

Y ou have been told you have cancer. You have been told you need treatment. Your mind is a whirlwind of thoughts as you grapple with your treatment options. Your oncology team will be mapping out a plan for you, but your active participation in the process is important. This is your body and this is your life. Asking the right questions will help you understand your options and make decisions that are in your best interest. And know that you do have options. Weigh quantity and quality of life. If you are not comfortable with the treatment plan that has been mapped out for you, seek a second opinion. Now, more than ever, you need to put on that superhero cape and empower yourself to be proactive and prepared. You are your own best advocate.

Questions To Ask Your Oncologist

What type of cancer do I have? What organs are involved?

- Treatment will be based on the cell type and the organ(s) involved. You may have had a biopsy when cancer was suspected. With a biopsy, a sample of tissue, or in some cases the entire tumor is surgically removed and sent to a pathology lab in order to determine whether it is benign or malignant. A benign tumor is non-cancerous. A malignant tumor is one that can invade other tissue and is considered to be cancer. If malignant, the cells are studied to determine the type of cancer.

- Once the type of cancer is known, additional tests may be done that will help determine the treatment plan. Some tumors may demonstrate a genetic abnormality that can be targeted with specific treatments. Some cancer cells secrete tumor markers. Tumor markers are substances that the body, or the cancer itself, may release in response to cancer. Not all cancers have tumor markers, but if a tumor marker is elevated, it may help in making a diagnosis and it may be used to monitor treatment response or recurrence.

What is my stage?

- Oncologists stage cancer, usually with a numerical system, to indicate how big a tumor is and if it has spread to lymph nodes or distant organs. By knowing the stage, the oncologist can look at treatment guidelines and search for clinical trials that are specific to the type and stage of cancer you have. A cancer that is *Stage 0*, or *in-situ*, may require surgery and/or radiation. A tumor that has spread to lymph nodes or distant organs may require chemotherapy, in addition to surgery and/or radiation therapy.

- *Stage 0 or In-situ:* Abnormal cells detected in an organ is often called dysplasia. This type of tumor is non-invasive but could become an invasive cancer if left to grow. Surgery and/or radiation may be ordered.

- *Stage I:* The tumor is small and contained in a single organ.

- *Stage II:* The tumor is larger than Stage I and it may have spread into the lymph nodes close to the tumor.

- *Stage III:* The tumor is large and has spread to lymph nodes and possibly tissue that is close to the original tumor site.

- *Stage IV:* The cancer has spread to areas distant from the original tumor site. This is *metastasis.*

What is the goal of treatment?

- *Cure:* Treatment is aimed at annihilating all the cancer cells and achieving remission.

- *Stabilize:* Treatment is aimed at slowing the growth of cancer cells to prevent the cancer from spreading.

- *Palliation:* If cancer is in an advanced stage, treatment may focus on controlling symptoms and providing comfort and quality of life.

What treatment is recommended? What are my options?

- *Conventional Treatment:* This is also known as allopathic treatment, Western medicine, or standard treatment. It is focused on the diagnosis and treatment of illness and disease and is administered by a healthcare professional. Conventional medicine includes surgery, chemotherapy, radiation therapy, immunotherapy, and biotherapy.

- *Clinical Trial:* Clinical trials help determine whether a new drug has benefits beyond current treatment, what types of cancer may respond, and what side effects can be expected.

- *Integrative Medicine:* This is a holistic type of medicine that focuses on mental, physical, emotional, and spiritual aspects of a person. It combines complementary or alternative treatment with conventional treatment.

- *Complementary Therapies:* Complementary therapy refers to the use of healing products or therapies that address the mind-body connection. Examples include yoga, aromatherapy, reiki, and therapeutic touch.

- *Alternative Treatment:* This treatment refers to therapies used in place of conventional treatment. An example may be a special diet or the use of a supplement in place of chemotherapy. If you decide to pursue alternative treatment, consider safety and potential side effects. Conventional treatments must undergo rigorous clinical trial before being made available to the public. Alternative treatments do not undergo the same rigorous testing and their safety and benefits may not be addressed.

- If you are considering complementary or alternative treatment, a great resource is the National Center for

Complementary and Integrative Health found at www.nccih.nih.gov.

How often and how many treatments will be given? What will be the total duration?

- The answer to this question will depend on the treatment given and the goal of treatment.

How will the treatment be administered?

- The answer to this question also depends on the treatment given.

What side effects should I expect and how will it impact my daily life?

- The oncologist and the nurse will provide you with information about possible side effects. It would be impossible to mention every side effect for every treatment, so they will talk with you about those that are most common. No two people will respond the same way. Doctors and nurses use many medications and strategies to minimize or prevent side effects. See more about side effects in Chapter 8.

What is my risk of recurrence with treatment? What is my prognosis?

- The oncologist will provide you with your risk of recurrence and prognosis based on statistical data. Keep in mind that these are numbers based on studies of very large groups of people with similar cancers and similar treatments. These numbers may help you make a treatment decision, but they can't predict how you, the individual, will respond.

Understanding And Preparing For Treatment

Your treatment plan may include a single type or a combination of treatments. Whatever the plan, it will be specific to you. The oncology team will take into account your overall health, any other medical conditions you may have, your tumor cell type, the tumor cell genetics, tumor markers, and your stage. Just like no two individuals are exactly alike, no two cancers are exactly alike. You may talk with other cancer patients with a similar cancer and find that their treatment plan may have been a little different than yours.

Oncologists refer to guidelines established by the National Comprehensive Cancer Network (NCCN) to determine a treatment plan. The NCCN is comprised of 27 of the world's leading cancer centers that work together to develop treatment guidelines for specific cancers. These guidelines are based on research and help oncologists make decisions that will provide their patients with the best quality care.

NCCN has developed an easily used tool that allows patients to access the same guidelines that oncologists use to develop a treatment plan. These guidelines also include questions to ask your doctor, illustrations, a glossary, and fact sheets. You can access these patient guidelines at www.nccn.org.

Surgery

Once cancer is confirmed and the pathology report is obtained, surgery may become the next step in the treatment plan. These are three basic reasons for performing surgery:

1. *Curative surgery*: The tumor is removed in its entirety along with surrounding healthy tissue. The purpose of removing surrounding tissue is to decrease the chance that any stray cells are left behind. This is called obtaining *clean margins*. Suspicious lymph nodes, thought to contain cancer, may also be removed. Curative surgery may be the only treatment necessary, or it may be followed by chemotherapy, radiation therapy, immunotherapy, hormonal therapy, or a combination of these.

2. *Debulking surgery*: If the tumor is large, or it is located in an area that would make it difficult to remove in its entirety, the surgeon may opt to remove as much as possible. This makes treatment with chemotherapy or radiation therapy more effective.

3. *Palliative surgery*: Palliative surgery can improve quality of life when cancer is advanced or widespread. This procedure can help relieve pain or restore physical function when a tumor is causing pressure or blockage.

Questions to Ask About Surgery

- What is the goal of surgery?

- What type of surgery will I have?

- What are the risks and benefits?

- What should I expect during recovery and how long should it take to recover?

- How many of these surgeries do you perform each year? What is the success rate?

- What type of care will I need at home? Should I anticipate needing home health care?

- Will I need any special clothing to accommodate the dressing or drain(s)?

- What signs/symptoms should I report once I am discharged from the hospital?

Preparing for Surgery

- Consider getting a second opinion.

- Make sure both the surgeon and the facility are in-network.

- Purchase any special clothing you may need to make yourself comfortable after surgery, such as cotton t-shirts, spots bras, elastic-waist pants, and button-down tops.

- Treat yourself to new slippers, pajamas, and non-slip socks that will make you feel comfortable when you get home.

- If your bedroom is upstairs, prepare a comfortable area on the first floor while you recover.

- Prepare individual servings of meals in easy-to-heat containers.

- Have healthy, small snacks available in case you have less of an appetite after surgery.

- Keep important names and contact numbers in a clearly-visible place should you or your caregiver need these once home. Think about including your surgeon, primary care physician, home health care, pharmacy, and friend/family/neighbor.

- If you need to have a caregiver after surgery, make sure they understand what you will need.

- Consider addressing your advanced directives and naming a health care proxy before you are admitted for surgery. This will give you the opportunity to make choices regarding your medical care before surgery. The health care proxy will be the person you choose to oversee your wishes. For more information, go to www.caringinfo.org or www.cancer.net.

Radiation Therapy

Radiation therapy works by damaging and destroying cancer cells. It targets the tumor site, sparing surrounding tissue. Side effects are related to the area that is exposed to the radiation. Radiation therapy may be given after surgery or chemotherapy to destroy microscopic cancer cells that may remain. This is called *adjuvant treatment*. It may also be administered in order to shrink a tumor prior to surgery. This is called *neoadjuvant treatment*. Radiation may also be used as *palliative therapy* to shrink a tumor, reduce pain and symptoms of the disease, and improve quality of life.

There are many different ways to administer radiation. External beam radiation targets the tumor from the outside. Brachytherapy is internal radiation in which seeds, beads, wires, or catheters are inserted directly into the tumor site. Sometimes chemotherapy is given along with radiation to potentiate the effects of the radiation. Radiation therapy is usually given daily over several days or weeks.

Questions to Ask About Radiation Therapy

- What is the goal of radiation therapy?

- What is the benefit of radiation therapy when compared to other treatment modalities?

- How many treatments will I receive?

- How will the radiation be administered?

- What are the short-term side-effects? What are possible long-term side effects?

- How can I prevent/manage side effects?

- Should I wear any special types of clothing? What type of clothing should I avoid?

- Who should I call if I have questions or concerns?

Preparing for Radiation Therapy

- Make sure that the radiation oncologist and the facility are in-network. Consider proximity of the facility to work or home since radiation therapy is often given Monday through Friday.

- Ask to meet with the billing department or a navigator to find out what out-of-pocket expenses you can expect.

- Schedule treatments at a time that is convenient for you. If you work, you may want to consider having treatment later in the day so you can go home after.

- The initial visit with the radiation oncologist will be a consultation. Bring your buddy with you, if possible. Your medical history will be reviewed and your treatment plan will be discussed. This is a great time to ask all the above questions.

- After your consultation, you will have a simulation. The area to be treated will be mapped out. Expect to have a CT scan so the radiation oncologist can pinpoint the area that needs to be radiated and areas to be avoided. You may be fitted for a mold that will immobilize the area to be treated. Markings or tattoos may also be placed in the area of radiation.

- Treatment generally begins 1-3 weeks after simulation.

- Your radiation oncologist will meet with you once a week throughout your radiation treatment to check on your progress and address any questions or concerns.

- Make sure that you have any special clothing you may need before starting treatment.

- Ask what you can use on your skin to prevent redness or burning and have that on hand to use every day.

- If you will be having radiation to the head and neck or the abdominal area, eating and maintaining your weight during treatment may be difficult. Ask for a referral to a dietitian who can help you develop a plan to address your nutritional needs throughout treatment.

- If you will be having radiation to the head and neck area, swallowing may be difficult. You may need a feeding tube placed in order to maintain your nutrition throughout treatment. The feeding tube will be removed once you are able to demonstrate an ability to eat and maintain calories. Ideally, the feeding tube should be placed prior to starting radiation.

- Ask your radiation therapist who you should contact if you have side effects of treatment. You will also want to know if there are any medications that you should keep on hand.

- Expect the unexpected. At times treatment may need to be delayed or rescheduled. If you had planned a special event or vacation prior to starting treatment, let your radiation oncologist know.

Chemotherapy

Chemotherapy is the use of drugs, or a combination of drugs, which attack cancer cells systemically, meaning it affects your entire body system. Cancer cells grow and multiply without any brakes, eventually forming a tumor. Cancer cells can also travel throughout the blood stream or lymphatic system and take up residence in other areas of the body, or *metastasize*. Systemic therapy can be an important part of the treatment plan since it can kill tumor cells, as well as those cells that metastasize. These drugs can work by disrupting the processes that cancer cells use to divide, grow, multiply, and travel. Healthy cells also divide and multiply, which is why chemotherapy can cause side effects.

Goals of Chemotherapy:

- *Cure:* Destroy cancer by eradicating all cancer cells in the body, including those not visible to the eye.

- *Control:* When cure is not an option, chemotherapy can be used to slow cell growth and/or kill cells that have metastasized or spread.

- *Shrink:* Chemotherapy can help shrink large tumors, making surgery or radiation therapy easier. This is known as *neoadjuvant treatment.*

- *Palliate*: Chemotherapy can reduce or relieve symptoms of the disease. A tumor can press on a nerve or organ causing pain. It may press on the spine causing a loss of body function or put pressure on an organ, making digestion difficult. By shrinking the tumor, the symptoms are lessened.

Understanding Your Chemotherapy Treatment Plan

Chemotherapy, or chemo, is commonly administered by mouth or through a vein. A Port may be placed prior to chemotherapy to make administration safer and easier. A Port is a small disc with a catheter at the end, inserted by a surgeon under the skin. The catheter rests in a vein and, once inserted, the skin over the catheter heals and the Port can be felt but it can't be seen. Ports eliminate the need for multiple needle sticks. They can be used for drawing blood for labs and for administering intravenous medications.

Chemotherapy may be given as a single-agent (one drug) or in combination with other drugs (regimen). Often you will hear chemotherapy regimens referred to by an acronym that stands for the drugs that make up that regimen. For instance, FOLFIRI stands for FOLinic acid, Fluorouracil (5FU), and IRInotecan. R-CHOP stands for Rituxan, Cyclophosphamide, Hydroxydaunorubicin, Oncovin, and Prednisone. It's a good idea to have the oncologist or chemotherapy nurse write down the names of your chemotherapy regimen so you can keep it in your records.

Chemotherapy is given at a scheduled frequency over the course of several months. This gives the chemotherapy the best chance of killing as many cancer cells as possible as they divide and grow. Each treatment is called a *cycle*. Since chemotherapy can also affect normal, healthy cells, a break is given between cycles to allow the healthy cells time to recover.

If you are considering having children in the future, ask the oncologist how you can preserve your fertility. Chemotherapy can cause infertility and it can put women into a temporary menopause and lower the sperm counts in men. Talk with your oncologist *before* you start treatment. Live Strong has a fantastic website, www. fertilehope.org, that may be helpful in understanding options.

Questions to Ask About Chemotherapy

- What is the goal of the chemotherapy?

- What will I be receiving? How will it be administered?

- How often will I receive treatment? How long will I be receiving treatment?

- What are the potential side effects? What side effects are short-term and what side effects may be long-term?

- Who should I call if I am not feeling well after hours?

- Will I be given prescriptions in case I do not feel well?

- How do I prevent/manage potential side effects?

- How often will I see the oncologist?

- How will I know if the chemotherapy is working?

Preparing for Chemotherapy Treatment

- Make sure that the cancer treatment center is in-network.

- Ask to meet with the billing department, navigator, or social worker to find out what out-of-pocket expenses you can expect and what resources may be available to you.

- Ask for a referral to a dietitian who can help develop a nutrition plan to make sure you meet your nutritional requirements throughout treatment.

- Schedule treatments at a time that is convenient for you. If you work, you may want to consider having treatment later in the day so you can go home after.

- Wear comfortable clothes.

- If the oncologist feels you need to have a ride to/from treatment, plan ahead. Driving yourself is usually okay, but at times having transportation is best. You may want to consider friends, family, or a neighbor. The American Cancer Society may be able to assist in coordinating transportation. You may also find assistance from your area's Department of Senior Services or through a religious organization.

- Put together a chemotherapy bag that includes books, cards, music, a laptop or tablet, a pillow, blanket, water, and healthy snacks.

- Every drug has its own set of side effects. That does not mean that you will experience any or all of them. Every person reacts differently. Plan ahead, though. If your chemotherapy nurse advises you to take medication to prevent side effects, do follow those instructions.

- Keep important numbers in a clearly visible place. Make sure you have the number for your oncologist or cancer treatment center on hand should you need to call after hours.

- If you have not done so already, call your insurance company to find out if they offer an oncology case management program. Ask to be assigned a case manager who will call you throughout your treatment and may be able to offer tips, suggestions, and support.

- Rev up your nutrition before, during, and after chemotherapy. This can be a challenge because chemotherapy may alter your taste, especially for foods that you normally enjoy. Your cravings for certain foods may increase, or may leave you with a decreased appetite. If the option is available, ask your oncologist for a consult with a dietitian or nutritionist. Plan ahead with easy to prepare healthy snacks and meals.

- Drink! Drink! Drink! You want to flush the chemotherapy out of your system and you do not want to get dehydrated. Avoid sodas and sugary drinks, as they can upset your stomach and can elevate your blood sugar. If you must have something sweet, try adding a bit of fruit juice to a glass of water or seltzer.

- Since chemotherapy can affect your immune system, complete any needed dental work before starting treatment.

- Get a calendar, planner, or use your smart phone to keep track of appointments Many people find that memory, concentration, and focus are not quite as sharp during chemotherapy treatments. We call this *chemo brain*. We really don't know how or why this happens, but it can last for a few months after treatment.

- Expect the unexpected. Treatment may not always follow the planned schedule. Treatment may be delayed or schedules changed for several reasons. If you have an event you wish to attend, or have made vacation plans prior to starting chemotherapy, let your oncologist know so you can work around your event or vacation.

Immunotherapy And Targeted Therapy

Cancer treatment is advancing much faster than ever before. It used to take more than 10 years for a drug to go through development and move to the clinical setting. That is changing. In the last two to three years, approximately 23 new drugs have been introduced to help treat cancer. This is due to clinical trials and the patients who participate in them.

Targeted therapy and immunotherapy are being used more frequently as part of the chemotherapy regimen, but they work differently than traditional chemotherapy. Targeted therapy involves the administration of a drug that blocks the cancer cell's ability to grow, divide, and multiply by targeting specific genes and proteins on the cancer cells. Targeted drugs are specific to the particular cancer cell. A tumor must possess the specific target or gene mutation in order for the drug to work.

Immunotherapy is the use of drugs that amplify one's own immune system. The immune system is put on overdrive so it can recognize and kill foreign invaders—cancer cells—in the body. Immuno-therapy drugs are fairly well tolerated but they do have side effects. Because the immune system is on overdrive, these drugs can induce an auto-immune response in the body, where the body recognizes its own cells as being foreign.

Clinical Trials

We would not be where we are today without clinical trials and the patients who participate in them. Over the past few years, we have seen developments and advances that are transforming the way we treat cancer, like the immunotherapy and targeted therapy drugs mentioned above. Clinical trials help determine whether a new drug has benefits beyond current treatment, what types of cancer may respond, and what side effects can be expected.

Clinical trials occur in stages, or phases:

- Phase I trials assess the safety and optimal dose of a drug or treatment.
- Phase II trials test the effectiveness of the drug or treatment on certain types of cancer.
- Phase III trials compare the new drug or treatment with current standard treatment.

A clinical trial may be an option if your cancer has progressed through previous treatment or you have advanced disease. But it may also be an option if you are newly diagnosed. By participating in a clinical trial, you may have access to new treatments that would not otherwise be available. Patients who participate in clinical trials receive close supervision at leading medical facilities.

There may be side effects, but a system is in place to closely monitor and manage participants.

Questions to Ask About Clinical Trials
- What is the goal of the clinical trial? What phase is the clinical trial?

- How will the treatment be administered and how often?

- Will I need to travel for the treatment or can it be administered close to home?

- What are the potential side effects?

- Who should I call if I am not feeling well after hours?

- Will I be given prescriptions in case I do not feel well?

- How often will I see the oncologist?

- How will I know if the clinical trial is working?

Talk to your oncologist if you are interested in finding out about clinical trials. You can also access the U.S. National Institutes of Health's website, www.clinicaltrials.gov, which contains information about clinical trials and allows you to search for trials based on your diagnosis and stage. Or call 1-800-4-CANCER to speak with someone who can help you in your search.

Hormone Therapy

Hormones are substances produced by your endocrine glands. They act as the body's messengers, sending information from one part of the body to the other. They regulate most major biological functions, such as hunger, blood sugar levels, sleep, and reproduction. Some cancers feed off of the body's hormones. Hormone therapy, also called *endocrine therapy*, works by blocking the particular hormone that feeds the cancer. This may be in the form of a pill or injection. Surgery may also be used to remove the organ that produces the offending hormone. Prostate cancer and breast cancer are two cancers that are often treated with hormone therapy.

The decision to take hormone therapy is something that your oncologist will discuss with you. During this discussion, you will want to ask about benefits versus risks. More specifically, you may want to ask what the risk of recurrence is with and without the hormone medication.

Stem Cell And Bone Marrow Transplant

Sometimes treating patients with very high doses of chemotherapy or radiation is necessary. These high-dose treatments are meant to wipe the body clean of cancer cells. But in doing so, the bone marrow can be destroyed. Without bone marrow, a person can no longer make white blood cells, red blood cells, or platelets. These cells are necessary for fighting infections, carrying oxygen and iron, and clotting the blood.

Stem cells are immature cells that become your body's blood cells (white blood cells, red blood cells, and platelets) and immune cells (lymphocytes). They are found in the bone marrow, circulating blood, and umbilical blood. A bone marrow transplant (BMT) or stem cell transplant (SCT) involves the transfer of healthy bone marrow or stem cells into the body so the bone marrow can regenerate. This treatment is commonly used to treat leukemia, lymphoma, and multiple myeloma. It is most effective when the cancer has already been put in remission.

In an *autologous* transplant, a person's own stem cells are collected and stored. They are reinfused after the person is treated with high-dose chemotherapy or radiation. In an *allogeneic* transplant, stem cells are collected from a donor, usually a family member or person whose stem cells closely match the patient's own stem cell make-up.

If you are a candidate for transplant, your oncologist will refer you to a transplant center for a consultation. Be sure to confirm that the transplant center is in-network prior to the consultation. Your insurance company will have a list of in-network transplant centers. Most insurance companies have transplant coordinators that will work with you, the referring oncologist, and the transplant center to coordinate your care. When choosing a transplant center, you may want to consider proximity to home, as you and your caregiver will need to stay near the facility for several weeks after the actual transplant. Your insurance company will be able to tell you whether you have travel and lodging benefits.

The initial consultation with the transplant team is very comprehensive. Bring your buddy for a second set of ears. You will meet with an oncologist who specializes in transplants, and with a transplant nurse who will explain the process to you in detail. The transplant team will assure that you are well-prepared and that all of your questions are answered.

Active Surveillance

Active surveillance may be the option of choice. If a cancer is slow growing, such as early stage prostate cancer, it may not warrant immediate treatment until the cancer shows signs of growing or progressing. Active surveillance may also be an option for those who have minimal disease that is not causing any symptoms. You may ask why someone would opt for no treatment when they know they have cancer. The fact is that there may be less of a benefit in treating a dormant or slow growing cancer. So, instead, the oncologist will keep a very close eye by developing a schedule of blood work and scans so that treatment can be initiated if the cancer begins to grow.

How Will You Know If The Treatment Is Working?

Your oncologist will meet with you on a regular basis to monitor your progress. You will have a physical exam and possibly blood tests. If your tumor produces tumor markers, your oncologist may check the level periodically through a blood test. If the level decreases or returns to normal during treatment, that would indicate a positive response to treatment. If the level increases, your oncologist will decide whether treatment needs to be changed. Your oncologist may also order scans such as a CT, MRI, or PET. The scans will be compared with any previous scans you had and will help determine response to treatment. Ask your doctor how your particular cancer will be monitored.

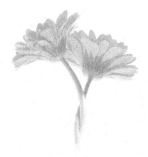

Part II

Caring for Your Mind

Chapter 4

Nurturing Your Spirit

Now that you have completed five of the six steps from your checklist and have a better understanding of your insurance, benefits, and treatment options, it's time to focus on you. Do not let cancer define you. A cancer diagnosis is no excuse for letting your health go. Now, more than ever, the health of your mind, body, and spirit is of the utmost importance. You need strength to help you heal. You need to care for your emotions and spirit to create wellness. Mind, body, and spirit go together and they function better together.

In this chapter, you will learn ways to nurture your spirit and help you cope. Mind-body modalities will be addressed to help you foster a sense of well-being. Later chapters will focus on stress and depression, nutrition, side effects, intimacy, quality of life, and planning for the future.

Cancer can take your sense of control away. You did not write this script. But you can be the director and choose how this script is played out. By nurturing the mind, body, and spirit, you can regain control and choose how you want to live.

Facing an illness can feel like someone stuck a pin in your heart and deflated your spirit. The response may be to grab hold of your faith and feel a closer religious connection. Or you may question your faith, values, and beliefs. These reactions are normal. No matter what you are feeling or experiencing, don't neglect your spiritual side. The spirit connects the mind and body. It makes you whole. By addressing spirituality, you can find comfort, support, and meaning.

Before moving on, there is a difference between being *religious* and being *spiritual*. You do not need to be religious to be spiritual. Many people interchange the terms, but they do have different meanings. Religion is a set of beliefs and practices within an organized group. Spirituality is a person's sense of purpose and a belief that there is a power greater than oneself. It is a feeling of being connected to self, nature, and others. It's what gives purpose and meaning to life. It may be different for each of us.

Spirituality and the Cancer Journey

People with a strong religious or spiritual identity report better overall health and wellbeing. Religious and spiritual people adapt better to stressful life situations and cope better with illness. Spiritual practices benefit mental and physical health in such a way that they can positively impact physical health and response to treatment. It is not only the physical actions of praying and going to church, but one's faith and spirituality that have been identified as having a strong impact on health.

Spirituality can have the following effects:
- Improved sense of physical wellbeing
  - Decreased anxiety, depression, anger, and discomfort
  - Improved pain control, decreased nausea, and decreased blood pressure
- A sense of inner peace
  - A feeling of belonging and community
  - Increased ability to enjoy life
  - Enhanced hope and optimism
- Enhanced coping skills

Finding Spirituality

Take a look at the following questions. How would you answer them? Your response will bring awareness to your values and your spirituality.
- What gives my life meaning?
- What gives me a sense of purpose?
- What helps me connect with others?
- What connects me to nature?
- How do I connect with myself?
- What do I value?
- What brings me peace? Joy? Love?

Stress Reducers and Happiness Inducers

Consider these suggestions for bringing more spirituality, peace, and comfort into your daily life:

- *Meditation, guided imagery, and breathing exercises:* These activities can be used anytime and anywhere to decrease anxiety and create a sense of calm. We will address this in more detail in the following chapter.

- *Pray, read scripture, attend a religious service.*

- *Music:* Listen to music, sing, or play an instrument.

- *Art therapy:* Drawing, painting, sculpting, or even coloring in a coloring book can be therapeutic.

- *Write:* Keep a journal, write poetry, blog, or create a short story.

- *Nature and sunlight:* Immerse yourself in nature. Sunlight helps to release serotonin from the brain. Serotonin is a chemical that helps boost mood, enhance creativity, and increase focus. Just remember to wear sunblock and a wide-brimmed hat.

- *Laugh:* Watch a funny movie. Read a funny book. Spend time with friends and loved ones. Some communities are now offering laughter yoga classes, so check out your local yoga studio or hospital wellness center.

- *Hobbies:* Set aside time for an activity that you have enjoyed in the past.

- *Pets:* Pets provide love, comfort, and can encourage you to get outside.

- *Essential oils:* Essential oils can be mood boosters. Lavender, bergamot, ylang ylang, and citrus oils such as lemongrass, sweet orange, and grapefruit have been shown to alter the body's chemistry to increase energy, create calm, and reduce stress and anxiety. Place a drop or two in the palm of your hands and rub together. Now inhale. Another way to enjoy essential oils is through a diffuser or by placing a few drops in a carrier oil, like almond or grapeseed, then massaging into your skin.

- *Move*: Get your body moving. Dance, walk, or swim. Try tai chi or yoga. Physical activity helps to release chemicals called endorphins. Endorphins help improve immunity, reduce sensations of pain, and are natural mood boosters.

- *Positive mantras*: Keep a list of positive sayings or funny sayings. You can put them on sticky notes and stick them in places where they will be visible to you, such as a bathroom mirror, the refrigerator, the car dashboard. Repeat them when you need to be lifted. Use them to replace negative thoughts.

- *Touch therapy*: You may want to give therapeutic touch, reiki, or reflexology a try.

- *Eat well:* Foods rich in omega-3 and folic acid are good for the brain. Try salmon, avocado, spinach, and flax seed oil.

- *Mindfulness*: Meditation, guided imagery, and breathing exercises can be used anywhere and anytime to decrease anxiety and create a sense of calm. Because mindfulness has tremendous benefit, we will discuss it in more detail.

Mindfulness

Another way to bring further peace and comfort into your life is through the practice of mindfulness. Most of us go through life like worker bees. Our minds flit from one thought to the next like a bee buzzing from flower to flower. We lay in bed, thoughts swirling, unable to rest. The worker bee goes through life fluttering from flower to flower, never stopping to soak in the beauty—never stopping to live in the moment.

When confronted by cancer and illness, fear, passivity, and loss of control can easily take over. The challenge is in stopping the mind chatter. But, unlike the worker bee, you have the ability to slow down and find contentment. You don't need to see cancer as something that controls your life or something to endure. You can learn to free yourself from the swirling thoughts and find peace within. No matter how stressed, overwhelmed, or restless you feel, you have the power to unleash yourself from the mindless chatter.

One of the best things you can do for yourself is to learn how to clear your mind and become grounded. In doing so, you can gain more control and empower yourself to meet your diagnosis head on and live each day in the moment. The practice of mindfulness can help take you to a place where illness and suffering don't exist. It can take you to a place where you can focus and find clarity.

By learning how to live in the moment, you will become stronger, resilient, and at peace with yourself. You will begin to feel a connection with spirit, mind, and body—a sense of oneness. When the mind is healthy, the body follows. This sensation of oneness—of wholeness—can transcend thoughts and feelings. Have you ever looked at the ocean, a sunrise, or a mountain and felt an overwhelming sense of awe? It is this sensation that can be achieved by practicing mindfulness. Mindfulness creates positivity, leaving less room for negative thoughts and feelings.

Mindfulness is a way of quieting the mind chatter by bringing awareness to the present moment. It provides a doorway for relaxation, compassion, resourcefulness, and gratefulness to enter your life. When dealing with cancer, you need all the resources available to help you stay focused and grounded during every phase of your cancer journey. Mindfulness helps you tune into yourself so you can find peace and resiliency, especially when you are suffering.

Cancer can be physically and mentally debilitating. For many, there is a sense of disorder and a loss of control. There may be a sense of fear. Mindfulness practices take you to a place where fear and illness do not exist. You gain control simply by letting go.

Achieving Mindfulness Through Meditation

Meditation has both physical and mental health benefits. Creativity and focus are enhanced and the mind feels calm and peaceful. People who practice meditation on a daily basis report being happier, healthier, and content.

Cancer patients who practice meditation on a consistent basis have reported better sleep, decreased depression, and decreased pain sensation. Meditation has been found to increase the brain's gray matter which leads to decreased pain sensitivity and an enhanced immune system.

So what's stopping you from considering meditation?

- *I don't have time.* It takes just 5-10 minutes of quieting the mind to reap the benefits of mindful meditation and it can be practiced in almost any setting.

- *I can't quiet my mind.* That's okay, and that's the point of mindful meditation. It creates an opportunity to recognize thoughts and feelings and creates room for contentment.

- *This sounds like some hippy stuff.* Mindful meditation is not about escaping reality. It's about quieting the mind and finding peace among all the cluttered thoughts. When the mind is clear, you are better able to focus and be courageous. So, maybe the hippies were on to something.

- *Isn't meditation a religious thing?* Although there are religions that practice meditation, it is not a religion or faith-based practice. It is fitness for the mind, plain and simple. Our minds and bodies are connected. So it stands to reason that a healthy mind facilitates wellness.

Mindful Meditation in Three Simple Steps

1. **Find a comfortable position**. You can sit or recline. Use pillows as props, if needed. Eyes can be open or closed. Hands can be on the belly or chest.

2. **Focus on your breath**. Breathe naturally. Notice the nourishing "in" breath. Notice the cleansing "out" breath. Some people find it helpful to silently repeat a phrase such as, "I am strong. I am grounded."

3. **When your mind wanders, draw attention back to your breath.** Let go of judgment. You can begin again and again. Herein lies the beauty of this practice.

There are several apps for smart phones, tablets, and personal computers that provide guided meditations. Insight Timer provides thousands of guided meditations, music tracks and talks that facilitate a daily mindfulness practice. You can explore at www. insighttimer.com or download the free app for your smart phone. Headspace, www.headspace.com, provides instruction in meditation and Buddhify, www.buddhify.com, allows you to select themed meditations. Both are available on your computer, tablet, and smart phone. There may be a small fee if you wish to subscribe. Thisiskara, www.thisiskara.com, is also available for your smart phone, computer, or tablet. It was designed specifically for cancer patients and includes 12 tracks addressing the physical and emotional issues that cancer patients experience.

Achieving Mindfulness by using Breathing Exercises

Pranayama is the practice of controlling one's breath to clear emotional and physical obstacles. Breathing is something that is often taken for granted, something that is done organically. But when stressed, the body becomes tense, and breathing becomes heavy and rapid. Pranayama breathing exercises can help bring calm and peace to areas that feel congested and tense. The following exercises can help increase energy, facilitate restful sleep, and boost the immune system. They can be practiced anywhere and anytime you need to find balance and release tension.

Three Breathing Exercises to Try

1. **Equal Breathing**: This breathing exercise calms the mind, enhances focus, and helps with sleep.

a. Slowly inhale through the nose for a count of 4. (If breathing through the nose is challenging, you may do this exercise with mouth breathing).

b. Exhale through the nose for a count of 4.

c. Repeat until you feel calm and relaxed.

d. Once you feel comfortable with this exercise. Try holding the breath for a count of 4 after each inhale and exhale.

2. **Alternate Nostril Breathing:** This breathing exercise creates calm and balance and increases energy.

   a. Place your right thumb over your right nostril, and inhale through your left nostril.

   b. Close your left nostril with your ring finger and exhale through your right nostril.

   c. Inhale through your right nostril.

   d. Now close your right nostril with your thumb and exhale through your left nostril.

   e. Repeat the sequence.

3. **Progressive Relaxation Breathing:** This exercise relieves tension.

   a. Close your eyes and focus on tensing and relaxing each muscle group for 2-3 seconds while taking slow deep breaths.

   b. Start at the feet and toes.

c. Move up to the legs and knees.

d. Now tense and relax the thighs and backside.

e. Move to the chest.

f. Work your way down from the arms to the hands and fingers.

g. End with your jaw and eyes.

Using Guided Imagery to Achieve Mindfulness

Guided imagery is a form of meditation incorporating images and sounds, or music, to distract the mind and quiet the chatter. Like mindful meditation, guided imagery can be practiced anywhere. All it takes is the creation of a peaceful, safe, and beautiful mental image that allows you to detach from the negative thoughts and feelings. It can help decrease the unpleasant effects of cancer and treatment by increasing energy, motivation, and hope. Guided imagery can help stimulate the immune system by increasing the number of natural killer cells.

Guided Imagery Basic Steps

1. Find a comfortable place.

2. Close your eyes and take a few slow breaths.

3. Picture a beautiful, relaxing, joyful place. It could be a beach, a mountain, a room, any place that creates pleasure and tranquility.

4. Use your senses. What sensations do you feel? What sounds do you hear? What do you see?

5. Remain in this place as long as you like.

6. Return to this place whenever you want to or need to.

You can download guided imagery meditations with smart phone apps like Calm, www.calm.com, and Sattva, www.sattva.life/apps, available for both iPhones and androids. Both offer free guided meditations, as well as subscriptions to premium services.

Yoga and Mindfulness

Yoga brings together mindful meditation, breathing exercises, and physical activity. It is a wonderful way to bring mind, body, and soul together. The poses open up blocked energy and help keep the body supple. The breathing exercises cleanse the mind, decrease distractions, and increase mindfulness. Many yoga studios, hospitals, and cancer centers offer yoga for cancer patients. These classes are taught by instructors who have had advanced training in working with cancer patients. The instructors will know how to modify poses to make them comfortable for you. Restorative yoga classes incorporate props such as pillows, bands, and blocks to enhance comfort. If you are not able to find a class in your area, try ordering a video or searching YouTube.

Mind-body Practices

If cancer takes away your sense of control, mindfulness and spirituality can bring this control back by allowing time to reflect and find the healthy person within. When the mind is calm and relaxed, the body can focus on healing. Spiritual practices, meditation, guided imagery, pranayama, and yoga are mind-body practices that can help relieve depression, elevate mood, and decrease physical pain. By practicing mindfulness and spirituality on a daily basis, you give yourself permission to spend your *now* loving and laughing.

Chapter 5

Stress, Emotions, and Depression

Understanding Stress and Emotions

A cancer diagnosis can be overwhelming to you, your family, and your loved ones. You may be dealing with a whole host of emotions, like anxiety around test results and treatment. You may feel distressed as you think about your future, your life's goals and wishes. Family roles may change. Relationships may change. Employment and finances may be a concern. You may be dealing with grief or anger or questioning your faith or beliefs. All of these feelings are normal. Addressing spirituality and mindfulness and be challenging when you are trying to come to terms with your feelings.

There's no doubt about it—coping with cancer is stressful. But it's how you deal with this stress that counts as you travel this cancer journey. When exposed to a stressful situation, the body goes into fight-or-flight mode. Hormones called epinephrine and norepinephrine are released, which cause a rise in blood pressure, heart rate, respiratory rate, and blood sugar. Attention is focused on either fighting or fleeing the situation. When stress is unrelenting, and escaping is not an option, stress can have a negative impact. It can affect your digestive system, weaken your immune system, and affect your overall wellbeing. Not exactly what you want when you are trying to fight cancer.

Stress can lead to anxiety, a feeling of uneasiness, intense fear, or worry. Anxiety may be accompanied by physical symptoms such as headaches, fatigue, tension, achiness, shakiness, and racing thoughts. No clear evidence proves that stress causes cancer, but you can see how stress and anxiety can make it difficult to care for your mind, body, and spirit.

A major life change, like the loss of a job, divorce, a major move, or illness is stressful. Many people experience an initial period of grief before adjusting to the change. Disbelief, anger, shock, sadness, fear, loneliness, guilt, helplessness, and fatigue are common responses. Feelings and emotions are very personal and each of us experiences change and grief differently. Accept yourself and your feelings so you can gain clarity and move forward.

Tips to Help You Manage Stress

- Maintain a routine.
- Accept offers of help.
  - Ask for help when you need it. You may be surprised to find that friends and family are waiting to be told what

you need. Could you use help with errands, preparing meals, caring for a pet, carpooling your child?

- Set aside time for you.

  ◦ Set boundaries and limits.

  ◦ Communicate your needs.

- Have an emotional outlet, such as journaling, talking with friends/family, taking a walk, reading.

- Address your spirituality.

- Choose a mind-body practice that can become part of your daily routine.

- Join a support group in your community or online.

  ◦ The American Cancer Society (www.cancer.org) and your cancer treatment center can provide you with a list of support groups in your area.

  ◦ Cancer Support Community offers phone support at 1-888-793-9355 and online support at www.cancersupportcommunity.org.

  ◦ CancerCare offers counseling services and support at 1-800-813-4673 or online at www.cancercare.org.

- Write about your experience and your feelings.

  ◦ Keep a personal journal.

  ◦ Start an online journal or blog at www.caringbridge.org or Cancer Support Community's Life Line at www.cancersupportcommunity.org.

- Talk with a social worker, counselor, chaplain, or spiritual leader.

- Get help, guidance, and support with employment and work-related issues at www.cancerandcareers.org.

- Continue to set aside time for activities or hobbies that give you pleasure.

Knowing When You Need Help

There may be times when you feel stuck and find it difficult to move forward. You may experience overwhelming sadness, anger, and guilt. When this happens, depression can take over. This can zap energy, take away your drive and motivation, and leave you feeling empty. Not only that, but it makes it more difficult to nourish your body and mind and address your spiritual needs. Relationships may suffer. You may have more difficulty managing physical symptoms and treatment side effects. The first step to moving forward is identifying the problem and knowing when you need some help.

Being sad is different than being depressed. Being sad or having the blues is a normal emotion that is temporary and fades once you have adjusted to a situation. Depression is not a normal emotion. It is a mental illness that needs to be addressed and goes way beyond just being sad. It does not just go away. When someone is depressed, they lack motivation, joy, and happiness. There is a pervasive feeling of hopelessness. Life lacks meaning. Sadness may be a small part of depression, but some people who are depressed have no sense of emotion at all. They feel hollow.

Signs and Symptoms of Depression

- Ongoing sadness or feelings of emptiness
- Feelings of worthlessness or guilt
- Feelings of hopelessness
- Loss of interest in activities that were once enjoyable
- Decreased energy, fatigue, or sluggishness
- Difficulty focusing or making decisions
- Difficulty falling asleep, difficulty staying asleep, or wanting to sleep all day
- Change in weight, either from overeating or from loss of appetite
- Restlessness or irritability
- Thoughts of death or suicide

If you identify with two or more of these signs and symptoms, and they have lasted for two weeks or more, you may be suffering from depression.

Depression is nothing to be ashamed of. It is not a sign of weakness. It is a medical condition that needs to be addressed. You deserve to be happy. You did not ask for cancer and you did not ask for depression. Your emotional and spiritual health are just as important as the health of your body.

Healing Depression

You may find support in talking with a chaplain. A chaplain does not need to be of the same faith as you and they will not try to sway you to join their religion. Instead, a chaplain will help you work through your feelings and identify with your spirituality.

Another source of support can be a social worker or mental health counselor. Although family and friends may be available for comfort, it may be beneficial to speak with someone outside your immediate support network. Social workers and counselors have an objective ear and will not judge your feelings. They can teach you healthy coping methods, help you connect with support groups or resources, and serve as a sounding board for you to express your feelings. Many cancer centers offer social workers or counselors as part of their services, and often these services are free of charge. Cancer centers may also have support groups and chaplains available to their patients.

Many employers offer an Employee Assistance Plan (EAP). An EAP offers free, confidential short-term counseling services. Many insurance companies also offer behavioral health programs as part of their benefit package. Counseling is free and takes place by phone. These programs can also assist in finding a psychologist or psychiatrist in your area.

Let your health care provider know if you feel you are suffering from depression. Some treatments and medications can contribute to mood changes. Some cancer medications alter hormone levels and can cause mood swings. Steroids may be given to treat cancer symptoms or as part of the chemotherapy regimen, but these medications also cause mood elevations followed by irritability and sadness. Your oncologist can help determine whether your symptoms are related to the cancer treatment and can help devise a plan to address these symptoms. Your oncologist will also be able to refer you to a counselor who can work with you to help you feel better.

Antidepressant Medication

Perhaps counseling, spirituality, and mind-body practices aren't enough to be free you from the grasps of depression. When numbness sets in and nothing seems to clear the black cloud over your head, it may be time to think about medication. Remember, depression is not a sign of weakness that can be turned off with a switch. It is a medical diagnosis due to a chemical imbalance in the brain. Medication can help to create balance and help lift the black cloud. Many patients feel a great sense of relief after being placed on an antidepressant.

It may take several weeks for an antidepressant to begin working, and about 50 percent of people will report improvement within three months. Because these medications may take a while to begin working, be sure to continue with counseling, supportive care, and any spiritual practices that have been helpful. Psychotherapy and antidepressants complement each other and can offer the most benefit.

Talk with your oncologist or oncology nurse practitioner about your depression. They may feel comfortable treating your depression or may send you to your primary care physician or a psychiatrist who can oversee your mental health treatment. If you do receive a prescription from someone other than your oncologist, inform your oncologist because some cancer treatment regimens and antidepressants may overlap or interfere with each other. Your oncologist or oncology nurse practitioner can work with your prescribing physician to ensure your treatment plan is the best one for you. Sometimes it takes trial and error before finding the medication that works best. Although antidepressants are not addicting, you may need to take the medication for up to six months after you start feeling better.

Moving Beyond Stress

Stress is an inevitable part of life. It can affect both physical and emotional health. By addressing feelings and emotions, and taking steps to manage stress, focusing becomes easier. Be kind to yourself and do not let cancer define you. Utilize the resources available to you to help you move beyond stress. You deserve to be happy.

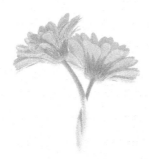

Part III

Caring for Your Body

Chapter 6

Make Nutrition
Your Prescription

In previous chapters, we talked about nourishing the mind and the soul. Now it's time to talk about nourishing the body. Cancer treatment is focused on killing malignant cells, but healthy cells can be damaged at the same time. This can have an impact on your immune system, digestive system, and your strength and stamina. Your body is battling this disease and needs to be armored to fight.

When dealing with cancer, everyone seems to have an opinion as to what you should or shouldn't eat. Family and friends may be giving you their opinions. Your physician may have told you to eat whatever you feel like during cancer treatment. Or maybe your physician has not mentioned nutrition at all. The internet is full of information on diets that claim to fight cancer, while advertisements for nutritional supplements are prevalent.

The incidence of obesity, diabetes, and cancer are rising, and an unhealthy diet is a big contributor. Supermarket shelves are stocked with boxes, cans, and packaged foods that look appealing, but may not have nutritional value. Canned nutritional drinks do not always have the most wholesome ingredients either. Eating "anything and everything" is not sage advice when fighting cancer. What do you do when you are bombarded with so much conflicting information?

Your oncologist has prescribed a treatment plan and has given you prescriptions to help manage side effects. One prescription you can give yourself helps you control your body and equip you to fight and mend. That prescription is nutrition. Nutrition is powerful stuff. It can positively or negatively affect tolerance to treatment and your quality of life. Nutrition can help strengthen the immune system, rejuvenate damaged cells, and contribute to healing.

Mother Nature provides all the nutritional resources the body needs. No fancy diet or expensive supplements needed. The best thing you can do for your body is to eat whole foods.

Whole Food

Whole food is Mother Nature's gift. Eating whole food means eating close to the ground—food that is in its natural, or very close to its natural, state. Whole food is minimally processed and refined, with little, if any, additives.

Plants contain phytonutrients called macronutrients and micronutrients. Think of macronutrients as the gas that makes our engines run—protein, carbohydrates, and fats. Think of micronutrients as the oil that keeps our engines running. This includes calcium, potassium, selenium, zinc, and vitamins like C, E, and A, to name a few. Phytonutrients are essential in keeping the body's engine running smoothly. Different foods contain different amounts of these goodies and they all work together. Plants also contain antioxidants that help fight the effects of stress on the body.

Whole Food Habit

The food we eat can heal us without any adverse effects. It can transform our health. The word *diet* dates back to the thirteenth century and literally means *a way of life*. The word has evolved over time and now it is associated with eliminating or giving something up. Nutrition should not be about elimination. It should be about giving the body what it needs to nourish itself. Nutrition should be about eating delicious, colorful foods that help sustain your body. It should be a way of life.

The whole food habit is not about elimination, it is about creating new habits that become integral to your daily life. It is about eating foods that are the way Mother Nature intended them—close to the ground, unprocessed, and in their natural state. When the focus is on eating more of the good stuff your body needs, there becomes less room for the things your body doesn't need. As you nourish your body, it begins to crave what it needs. Good nutrition leads to more energy and a more robust immune system—important stuff when it comes to fighting cancer.

The Five Parts Of Whole Food Nutrition

1. Fruits and Vegetables

Flood your body with fruits and vegetables. The more colorful the plate, the better it is.

- Choose colorful vegetables
  - Green: kale, spinach, collards, turnip greens, broccoli
  - Orange/yellow: sweet potatoes, orange peppers, winter squash, carrots
  - Red: tomatoes, beets, red potatoes, red peppers
  - Blue/purple: purple cabbage, eggplant
  - White: cauliflower, mushrooms, turnips, parsnips
- Choose colorful fruit
  - Green: kiwi, honeydew, green grapes
  - Orange/yellow: apricots, cantaloupe, nectarines, tangerines
  - Red: cherries, cranberries, pomegranates, strawberries
  - Blue/purple: blueberries, grapes, blackberries
  - White: bananas, white peaches, pears
- Tips:
  - Fresh is best, but frozen fruits and vegetables are fine and are more economical. Frozen products also reduce waste and tend to be easier to prepare.
  - Toss cut-up fruit into a blender with a handful of spinach or kale. Add coconut water, yogurt, and a splash of juice. Or try adding almond, cashew, soy, or coconut milk for a delicious smoothie.
  - Add frozen vegetables to pasta, baked potato, soup, or a scrambled egg for a quick, simple, and easy to digest meal.
  - Keep fruit salad and cut vegetables in the refrigerator for a quick snack.
- Note:
  - If your white blood count is low during cancer treatment, make sure you peel or cook your fruit and vegetables. Avoid berries and salads during this time.

2. Lean Protein

Protein is essential for growth and development. Your body needs protein to build muscle and strengthen the immune system. Most people get an adequate amount of protein in their daily diet. It can be more challenging for those undergoing cancer treatment because appetites may decrease, taste may change, and cooking may become trickier.

Many people tend to equate red meat with protein. Yes, red meat is protein, but it is not the only source of protein and certainly not the best source of protein. Plant-based proteins are easy to digest. They also provide a hefty dose of antioxidants to help protect and repair cells in the body. If you are craving a steak, burger, or pork chop, just make sure the meat you purchase is hormone-free and antibiotic-free. Avoid smoked or processed meat as these contain cancer-causing substances. Lean meats like chicken, turkey, and pork are alternatives to red meat.

Here is a short list of healthy protein-powered foods. If you have never tried some of the items below, now is the perfect time. These are all easy-to-digest protein sources and all are simple to prepare:

- Beans, legumes
  - Examples:
    - Chickpeas, lentils, red beans, fava beans, lima beans, and black beans.
  - Tips:
    - Add beans to soups.
    - Put them on top of a potato, rice, or noodles.

- Nuts, nut butters, and spreads
  - Examples:
    - Walnuts, peanuts, almonds, pistachios
    - Peanut, almond, or cashew butter
    - Hummus
  - Tips:
    - Hummus makes a great snack on toast or with whole grain crackers or vegetables.
    - Keep individual servings on hand for a quick snack.
    - Add nut butters to smoothies for extra calories and protein.
- Fish
  - Fatty fishes like salmon and tuna contain protein and healthy fats.
  - Lean fishes like halibut, cod, and snapper are great choices too.
- Seitan
  - This is a meaty-textured product derived from the protein portion of wheat. Seitan is not gluten-free, so avoid this if you have a gluten sensitivity.
  - Find it in the green section of your supermarket or in an organic or natural foods market.
  - Tip:
    - It is a great substitute for chicken or meat and is easy to digest.
- Quinoa
  - Quinoa is an ancient grain. It is gluten-free and one of the only plant-based complete proteins.

- Tips:
  - Prepare a batch, then add a splash of non-dairy milk, fruit, cinnamon, and raisins for a protein-packed breakfast.
  - Prepare it with broth and add it to salads, stews, or top it with beans and salsa.
  - Use it in place of rice.

- Seeds
  - Examples: Hemp seeds, chia seeds, flax seeds, pumpkin seeds, sunflower seeds
  - Tips: Seeds can be sprinkled on salads or added to yogurt or smoothies for extra protein.

- Eggs or egg whites

- Protein powders
  - Read the ingredient list before purchasing a protein powder. Many powders are on the market with varying lists of ingredients. You want one free of artificial colors or additives.
  - Plant-based protein powders are gaining popularity because they contain complete proteins, as well as fiber and anti-oxidants.
  - Whey protein is another option. Whey is a by-product of cheese production. Although it is considered dairy, it tends to be easier to digest than milk.

- Soy
  - Soy is fine in moderation. For years, people with thyroid issues and estrogen-positive breast cancer were told to avoid soy because it was thought to interfere with thyroid

function and increase estrogen production. Soy contains a substance called isoflavone. Although it is thought that isoflavones mimic estrogen, they actually block the receptors for estrogen, decrease the amount of estrogen in fat cells, act as anti-oxidants, boost the immune system, and decrease cancer growth. Studies have shown that soy can decrease disease recurrence in breast cancer survivors and soy does not interfere with thyroid function. The key is to ingest only non-GMO sources of soy and do so in moderation.

- Examples:
  - Tofu
  - Edamame (soy beans)
  - Tempeh (fermented soy beans)

- Tips:
  - Tofu on its own has very little flavor. It works well when cut in cubes and added to soups for a hefty dose of protein.
  - Tofu readily takes on the flavor of marinades. It can then be baked or pan-fried for a flavorful, soft, protein-packed meal.
  - Edamame can be found in the frozen section of the supermarket. You can purchase them in the pod or shelled. Simply cook in boiling water for 15 minutes, then eat as-is or add to salads or soups.
  - Tempeh is a nutty-textured fermented soy patty. You can find it in the green section of your supermarket or an organic or natural food store. It can be marinated and crumbled in chili or stew or baked and substituted for meat.

- Dairy
  - Dairy products contain protein, vitamin B12, vitamin D, potassium, and calcium—all necessary for building strong muscle and bones.

  - Examples
    - Milk
    - Cottage cheese
    - String cheese
    - Yogurt
    - Kefir

  - Tips:
    - There is a debate as to whether full-fat whole milk is better than low-fat milk, but the choice may come down to personal preference. Cow's milk may contain added hormones that may interfere with your hormone balance. To avoid this problem, choose milk that is labeled organic or rBGH-free.

    - Greek yogurt is lower in lactose, making it easier to digest for those with milk sensitivity. It also contains twice the amount of protein as regular yogurts. Yogurts contain probiotics that are beneficial to the digestive system. Since many flavored yogurts contain several grams of added sugar, try buying plain yogurt and adding fruit with a drop of maple syrup.

- Non-dairy beverages
  - Many people choose to avoid dairy products for a number of reasons. For those who are lactose-intolerant, dairy

products can be difficult to digest and may cause cramps and diarrhea. People following a vegan diet avoid all dairy, as well as meat, fish, and eggs. There is also an ongoing debate as to the role of dairy in decreasing or increasing the risk of certain cancers.

○ If you choose to avoid dairy products, there are many readily-available alternatives.

○ Many non-dairy beverages are fortified with calcium and vitamin D. Some are even fortified with vitamin B12 and protein.

○ Nut milks come in a variety of flavors, but those flavors may also mean added sugar and sweeteners. Opt for those that are labeled unsweetened.

○ Examples:
  – Almond milk
  – Soy milk
  – Rice milk
  – Cashew milk
  – Coconut milk
  – Hemp milk

3. Whole Grains

Whole grains contain the germ, endosperm, and bran. Refined grains, such as white rice, white flour, and white bread have been processed to remove the germ and bran. Whole grains contain fiber, B vitamins, antioxidants, and protein. The fiber in whole grains helps keep bowels healthy and moving. A diet rich in whole grains can reduce the risk of heart disease, diabetes, and obesity.

Whole wheat, rye, and barley are good sources of whole grain. For those concerned about gluten, the following whole grains are gluten-free:

- Millet
- Corn
- Buckwheat
- Oats
- Wild rice
- Brown rice
- Quinoa
- Grits
  - Tips:
    - Make a large batch of rice or quinoa to keep in the refrigerator for use throughout the week.
    - Add oatmeal to smoothies for increased fiber.
    - Grains can be topped with a protein and vegetable for lunch or dinner, or they can be topped with fruit and yogurt for breakfast or snack.

4. Healthy Fats

Fats serve as a source of energy and help transport vitamins A, D, E, and K through your bloodstream. Fats are essential for maintaining healthy hair and skin, repairing cell membranes, protecting the liver, and facilitating the development of the nervous system.

The human body is not able to produce all of the essential fatty acids that it needs, so it is important to eat a diet that can help supply them. Fats from plants and seafood are the best. Man-made, or hydrogenated fats, known as *trans fats,* are the least healthy. Fats from meat and dairy should be eaten in moderation.

Sources of healthy fats include:
- Wild salmon and tuna
- Chia seeds, flax seeds, pumpkin seeds
- Avocado
- Nuts
- Olive oil, coconut oil, and grapeseed oil

5. Probiotics

Probiotics are bacteria and yeasts essential for the functioning of your body. We often think of bacteria as being harmful, but your body is home to a large number of microorganisms that help digest food, fight disease, and produce vitamins. Cancer, antibiotics, diarrhea, obesity, and inflammatory bowel disease can create imbalance, impacting the amount of healthy microorganisms in the body. By eating fermented foods and yogurt rich in probiotics, you can restore balance to the digestive system, relieve diarrhea, and decrease inflammation. Antibiotics often cause diarrhea, as they kill bad, as well as good, bacteria in the body. Probiotics can be quite beneficial in preventing antibiotic-induced diarrhea.
- Examples:
  - Yogurt or kefir (a yogurt drink)
  - Miso soup
  - Pickles, sauerkraut, kimchi
  - Tempeh
- Tips:
  - Look for yogurt or kefir that states it contains live cultures.

- ◦ Many flavored yogurts have a high sugar content. Try plain yogurt and add fresh or frozen fruit.
- ◦ You can find miso paste in many organic or natural food markets.
- ◦ Add a tablespoon of miso paste to hot water to make a soothing drink. Add vegetables, noodles, and a protein and make it a meal.

Cancer Promoters

The foods listed in the previous pages are cancer fighters. They can help boost nutrition, the immune system, and overall wellbeing. Some foods can promote cancer when eaten in large amounts. The following is a list of foods that should be avoided or eaten in moderation:

- White sugar
- Boxed or processed foods
- Processed meats and cheeses
- Trans fats—These are man-made fats found in boxed and processed foods, as well as natural fats found in meat and some dairy products. Corn oil, canola oil, vegetable oil, margarine, and butter contain trans fats.

What's the scoop on sugar?

Not all sugar is bad. Naturally occurring sugar that comes from fruit, vegetables, and low-fat dairy is fine. Plus, naturally occurring sugars come with the added benefit of having vitamins and minerals. White sugar, sugar in the raw, and processed sugars, however, are broken down like alcohol, which is processed in the liver and is changed into fat. These sugars may be labeled as high-fructose corn syrup, agave nectar, evaporated cane juice, or fructose. Better choices would be honey, maple syrup, coconut sugar, or stevia.

Isn't fat healthy?

It is true that your body needs fat to maintain a healthy nervous system, but a diet high in trans fats and sugar can cause inflammation. Acute inflammation is beneficial because it initiates an immune response to help the body heal. But prolonged inflammation causes a host of problems in the body. When the body experiences prolonged inflammation, it becomes over-stressed and the immune system weakens. The body responds by decreasing resistance to insulin, which increases the risk for diabetes, dementia, cardiovascular disease, fibromyalgia, and cancer. Your body does not need added stress while trying to heal. Diets high in fat and sugar provide empty calories and little, if any, nutritional value. What is needed is food that will nourish and heal.

Nutrition Tips Before, During, And After Cancer Treatment

- Consult a registered dietitian who can assess your individual needs and develop a plan to help you get the most from your daily diet. A dietitian can also help address specific issues—diabetes, hypertension, nausea, and diarrhea—and give you tips to get through treatment.

- Better to eat small amounts every couple of hours than forcing yourself to eat three big meals. Small meals are easier to digest and may help stave off nausea.

- Keep your pantry stocked with nutritious foods that are easy to prepare. If you work, keep healthy snacks and plenty of water at your desk.

- Plan ahead for days when you do not have the energy or the time to prepare a meal. Freeze individual containers of soup, stew, or casserole so that you can grab and heat.

- Not sure how to get the most from your meals? Picture your plate as a smiley face. One eye is a serving of protein. The other eye is a serving of whole grain. The smile is your fruit and vegetables.

- Keep an insulated water bottle with you wherever you go. Keep track of how much you drink. Aim for eight cups of fluid each day.

- Don't like water? You can get fluids from grapes, oranges, broth, melon, and natural fruit popsicles. Try adding fruit or a splash of fruit juice to your water to give it flavor. Cucumbers add a refreshing taste. Lemon, lime, or orange slices can help freshen your mouth and keep it moist.

- Avoid fruit drinks and soft drinks which contain large amounts of sugar and empty calories.

Would you like more nutrition information? Check out Appendix B for additional tips and suggestions.

Chapter 7

Challenges to Eating Well

Y ou may hit obstacles on your cancer journey challenging your ability to eat well and nourish your body. Let's talk about some of the most common challenges you may face and how to manage them.

Increased Appetite, Cravings, Weight Gain

Some people are surprised to find that they gain weight during cancer treatment. There are several reasons for this. If you feel fatigued, you may be getting less physical activity. This lack of activity results in a slower metabolism and weight gain. Steroids given with many chemotherapy treatments can cause cravings, increased appetite, and fluid retention. Hormonal therapies are used to decrease estrogen and progesterone in women and testosterone in men. This decrease in hormones can slow metabolism and lead to decreased muscle tone and increased fat accumulation.

- Refer to the previous chapter focused on whole food nutrition. Review the tips and suggestions for nourishing your body.

- Stay well-hydrated, aiming for eight 8-ounce glasses of fluid per day. Water is best. You can try adding cut up fruit or cucumber to give it a refreshing taste. Fruit juices should be diluted with water, as they contain a lot of sugar. Avoid sugary drinks and sports drinks.

- If you are retaining fluid and your feet and ankles appear swollen, try elevating your feet when you are sitting. Decreasing salt intake helps. Avoid adding salt to foods and avoid eating canned or processed foods.

- Ask for a referral to a dietitian who can help you develop a plan to help manage your weight.

- Move your body. Take a walk, ride a stationary bike, use resistance bands. If you are overcome by fatigue, try seated exercises like leg extensions and arm curls with soup cans. No matter what you do, be consistent. Aim for a total of 30 minutes of activity at least 5 times per week.

- Stock your pantry with nutritious foods and keep snacks on hand, in the car, and at work. Avoid snack machines and fast food stops.

- Have a buddy who will motivate you to exercise and eat well.

- Programs such as www.myfitnesspal.com help you track what you eat and how often you exercise. These programs can help you make smart food choices and ensure that you are nourishing your body.

- Do not punish yourself if you give in to cravings. Sometimes it feels good to treat yourself. And if you eat well the majority of the time, an occasional treat really does feel like a treat.

Altered Taste and Smell

Chemotherapy, radiation therapy, and anesthesia used during surgery can affect your sense of taste and smell. Some people describe food as being metallic or having no taste at all. Some people find that foods take on a strong odor.

- Try eating foods that are cold or room temperature. Hot food tends to have a stronger odor and may be less appealing.

- Rinse your mouth with lemon water, alcohol-free mouth rinse, or a mixture of baking soda and water before eating. This can help clean your palate and moisten your mouth so foods taste better.

- Do not force yourself to eat foods that do not appeal to you. This only serves to create an aversion to those foods when you are feeling better.

- Experiment with spices and seasonings. Salt-free herb blends can bring out the taste of food.

- Avoid metal utensils if food has a metallic taste.

- Try marinades, gravy, sauces, or relishes to enhance the flavor of food.

- Lemon juice or vinegar can help decrease the metallic taste of foods.

- Cinnamon candies and lemon drops can increase saliva and decrease the metallic taste that may linger in your mouth.

Nausea

Nausea is a common side effect of chemotherapy and may occur with radiation therapy or after surgery. It may also be a symptom of the cancer itself. No matter the cause, nausea can greatly affect your ability to eat and enjoy your food.

- If you are receiving chemotherapy, talk with your physician or nurse so you understand how to take your anti-nausea or *antiemetic* medications.

- Focus on preventing nausea. Some people find it helpful to take their antiemetic medicine the night of chemotherapy and for a day or two after to prevent nausea.

- If you feel nauseas despite taking your prescribed medication, communicate with your physician or nurse. There are many options when it comes to antiemetics and one may work better for you than another. Antiemetics come in various forms. Some can be taken orally, others by suppository, some can be placed under the tongue, and others can be worn as a patch on the skin. Your physician can help find the one that works best for you. You don't need to suffer.

- This may sound counterintuitive, but it helps to eat something light every two hours. When the belly is empty, nausea tends to set in.

- Ginger works wonders for nausea. You can purchase ginger tea or cut a piece of fresh ginger root and steep it in a cup of hot water. Sip on this whenever you feel queasy. Ginger candies work well, too.
  - Note: Ginger should be avoided prior to surgery, or if you have a bleeding disorder, as it has anticoagulant properties. An alternative would be peppermint or chamomile tea.

- Try acupressure.
  - Use your thumb and index finger to apply pressure to the web of skin between the thumb and index finger of the opposite hand. Hold pressure for 3-4 minute intervals.
  - You also have a nausea acupressure point on your wrist. Place your first three fingers across your wrist until they are resting inside the two tendons below your thumb. Now use your thumb to massage the area for 3-4 minute intervals.
  - Most pharmacies sell acupressure wrist bands or motion sickness wrist bands that can be worn throughout the day to help relieve nausea.

- Peppermint, ginger, lavender, and chamomile essential oils help relieve nausea. Try placing a few drops on a tissue and carrying it with you.

Diarrhea

Diarrhea may be a side effect of chemotherapy, immunotherapy, radiation therapy, or the cancer itself. Diarrhea is defined as having three or more loose, watery stools in a 24 hour period. It may or may not be accompanied by abdominal pain and cramping.

Uncontrolled diarrhea can lead to dehydration and weight loss and can greatly impact quality of life. It can also affect tolerance to treatment. Let your physician know if you develop diarrhea. Treatment-related diarrhea needs to be addressed as soon as possible to avoid unnecessary complications.

- Your physician may instruct you to take an anti-diarrhea medication, such as loperamide (Imodium) at the start of diarrhea and after each loose bowel movement. If the loperamide does not control the diarrhea, contact your physician. You may need a prescription medication to help slow down the diarrhea.

- Talk to your physician about the possibility of receiving intravenous hydration, as this may help decrease the risk of dehydration.

- It may be necessary to hold your treatment until diarrhea resolves. Sometimes the dose of treatment needs to be decreased so you tolerate it better. This does not mean that your treatment will be any less effective. The oncologist needs to balance your treatment dose with your body's ability to heal itself between treatments.

- Drink plenty of clear liquids, such as broth, tea, water, diluted cranberry or grape juice.

- Avoid foods and beverages that can aggravate diarrhea. These include coffee, milk, spicy foods, fried or greasy foods, citrus fruits, and salads.

- Psyllium fiber found in bulk-forming laxatives is helpful for constipation. It can also help manage diarrhea. The psyllium absorbs water from the digestive tract and makes a bulkier stool.

- Try the BRAT diet to help slow diarrhea:
  - Bananas
  - Rice
  - Apple sauce
  - Toast.

- Once you have been free of diarrhea for 24 hours, you can start adding other foods into your diet. Stick with bland foods, such as potatoes, cooked carrots, noodles, eggs, hot cereal, and cooked squash. Then gradually increase portion size and foods, as tolerated.

- Probiotics restore the natural flora to the digestive tract, thereby helping the bowel return to its normal function. Yogurt, miso soup, and probiotic supplements can be very helpful for someone with diarrhea.

Mouth Sores, Dry Mouth, Difficulty Swallowing

Chemotherapy works by killing actively dividing cells, but it can't discriminate between cancer cells and healthy cells. The cells in the digestive tract divide rapidly and are often affected by certain chemotherapy drugs. The mucus lining of the digestive tract extends from the mouth, down the esophagus, through the stomach and intestines, and all the way to the rectum. That is why some people develop sores on the lips and gums. Others may develop a burning in the throat, irritation of the stomach, or exacerbation of hemorrhoids.

You may hear some various terms used to describe issues with the mouth and digestive tract: *Esophagitis* refers to inflammation of the esophagus or throat. *Stomatitis* is an inflammation of the mouth. *Mucositis* refers to inflammation of the mucus membranes lining the digestive tract. *Dysphagia* is a term used to describe difficulty swallowing or painful swallowing. *Thrush* is a fungal infection in the mouth, characterized by white patches or white coating on the gums or tongue.

Radiation therapy to the head and neck, or radiation therapy that involves any part of the throat, can cause inflammation and swelling, making swallowing difficult and painful. Radiation and chemotherapy can also cause dry mouth, making chewing and swallowing difficult.

- If possible, have a dental exam prior to starting treatment. If you have any dental issues, they can be taken care of before chemotherapy or radiation.

- Practice good oral hygiene throughout treatment. Use a non-alcohol mouth rinse at least twice each day. You can purchase one or make your own using one of the following recipes:
  - Mix 1 teaspoon baking soda in 1 cup warm water.
  - Mix ¼ teaspoon salt in 1 cup warm water.
  - Mix 1 cup hydrogen peroxide in 1 cup warm water.
  - Add a few drops of cinnamon or mint extract to any of the above recipes, if you like.

- Smoking can further irritate the lining of the mouth and throat. If you need help quitting, talk with your physician.

- Ask your chemotherapy nurse if you will be receiving any drugs that have the potential to cause mouth sores. If so, you can try sucking on ice chips while the chemotherapy infuses. The ice will slow the blood flow to the mouth and decrease the risk of mouth sores.

- Avoid spicy, acidic, or citrus foods that can burn the mouth.

- Avoid any dry or rough foods, and avoid any extreme temperatures.

- Smoothies, creamy soups, yogurt, avocadoes, eggs, noodles, and potatoes are bland, soothing, and packed with nutrients.

- Artificial saliva, moisturizing mouth sprays, sour candy, and sugarless gum can help with dry mouth.

- Use a water pick and soft-bristled toothbrush to clean your teeth and gums.

- Use moisturizer on your lips.

- If you develop an ulcer or sore in your mouth or on your lip, you can break open a vitamin E capsule and apply the oil, or you can swish and swallow two teaspoons of an over-the-counter antacid every three hours to decrease the burning. You can also use an over-the-counter topical coating agent for sores on the lips.

- Inform your physician of any oral discomfort. He or she may prescribe a solution that will numb the pain and heal the irritation, making it easier to eat and swallow.

Anorexia

Anorexia is a loss of appetite, or a decreased appetite, with weight loss. As we discussed in the previous chapter, good nutrition is vital to healing your body. But when your appetite is diminished, eating becomes a chore.

- Ask for a referral to a dietitian who can help you develop a plan based on foods that you enjoy eating.

- Create a pleasant atmosphere when you are eating. Play relaxing music and adjust the temperature in the room so you feel comfortable. Take the focus off the food.

- Eat every two hours. Try small plates and small portions.

- Eat foods that pack a punch. Smoothies, nut butters, potatoes and gravy, creamy soups are easy to get down and are nutrient-dense.

- Sipping is easier than chewing. Think about pureeing fruit and coconut milk in a blender. Or puree vegetables, broth, and a protein to make a soup.

- Exercise 30 minutes before you sit down to eat. It may perk up your appetite.

- Add mashed potato flakes to creamy soups, stews, and gravies to increase calories.

- Add yogurt or nut butters to shakes and smoothies.

- Purchase a protein powder to add to smoothies and shakes.

- Many health professionals encourage their patients to purchase canned nutritional supplements as a quick and convenient way to load up on calories. Most of these canned supplements have oil and corn syrup as the first ingredients—additives that can cause gas, bloating, and diarrhea. You can make your own nutritional drink by blending milk, yogurt, or non-dairy milk with fruit, greens, and protein powder. Homemade smoothies are delicious, nutritious, and much more economical.

- Try adding coconut oil, avocado, or full-fat coconut milk to soups or smoothies for a dose of healthy fat and calories.

- Lemon, lime, bergamot, ginger, peppermint, and spearmint essential oils can help stimulate appetite. Place a drop in your hands or on a cotton ball and inhale before eating. You can also try teas infused with those flavors.

- Discuss your lack of appetite with your physician. Several prescription medications are available that can help boost your appetite and make you look forward to eating.

Make Nutrition Your Prescription

Our culture puts much emphasis on food as being a source of pleasure. When cancer symptoms and treatment side effects get in the way of eating well, it can have a significant impact on you physically and mentally. Talk with your doctor or nurse about any issues you may be having that interfere with your ability to eat well. The National Cancer Institute offers a free publication, "Eating Hints: Before, During, and After Cancer Treatment." You can download the book by visiting www.cancer.gov and clicking on the *Publications* link. You can also order the book by calling 1-800-4-CANCER.

Chapter 8

Taking Control
of Side Effects

Cancer is a very personal experience. You may have been told the possible side effects of your treatment, but that does not mean that you will experience every one. Each person responds differently. Your physician and nurses will prepare you for treatment by providing you with a list of potential side effects and instructing you in ways to manage those side effects. Regrettably, no one can predict exactly what side effects will affect which patient.

Keep in mind that many side effects are preventable or manageable. Radiation side effects usually begin midway into treatment and can increase as treatment progresses. Chemotherapy side effects generally begin within a few days of treatment and begin to get better just before the next treatment is due. Some people find the side effects to be a mild nuisance and are able to go about their daily routine. Other people find some of the side effects to be distressing, impacting their ability to maintain their normal routine. Side effects are not an indication of whether treatment is working. If side effects become severe, the oncologist may change the dose or schedule of treatment to increase tolerability. This does not mean the treatment will be less effective.

Communication is the key to getting through your cancer treatment as smoothly as possible. Ask your nurse to write down specific instructions. If you do not understand something, ask for clarification. This is new territory and your needs and questions should be addressed. Ask what prescriptions you may need at home to manage potential side effects.

Keep your physicians' contact numbers on hand. If you are not feeling well or have concerns about medications or side effects, call the physician's office. All oncology offices have medical staff available after hours, on weekends, and on holidays. Managing a side effect is easier when it begins. Do not try to ride it out.

We talked about symptoms and side effects that challenge your ability to eat well in the previous chapter. This chapter addresses some of the other symptoms and side effects of cancer and cancer treatment, including tips for managing them. The most common symptoms and side effects are identified, as well as some of the medications and treatments that can cause these issues. But this is not meant to be an exhaustive list, so if you experience something that is not listed, but is a change from how you typically feel, report it to your physician or nurse.

A Few Words About Medical Marijuana

Because cannabis possession has been illegal in the United States, the topic has been taboo. But as its benefits for treating side effects are being documented, cannabis is getting more attention in the media and in the community. Before addressing specific side effects, the use of medical marijuana bears mentioning.

Cannabis contains substances called cannabinoids. The two most prevalent are THC and CBD. When smoked, vaporized, ingested, or applied topically, these substances bind to receptors in the brain and immune system and have the following benefits:

- Reduced pain sensation
- Relief from nausea and vomiting
- Increased appetite and increased weight
- Control of seizures
- Relief from anxiety
- Decreased inflammation
- Slowed growth of cancer cells

Dronabinol (Marinol) and Nabilone (Cesamet) are two manmade forms of THC that may be used to relieve nausea in cancer patients. They are available by prescription. Because they are manmade, they do not contain THC or CBD and lack the full benefits of cannabis.

Cannabis has the potential to enhance the quality of life for cancer patients, and this has spurred several states to discuss legalization. As of September, 2017, 29 states and the District of Columbia have enacted medical marijuana programs. Eligibility criteria and the laws regarding dispensing of medical marijuana vary by state and many health care professionals are not yet comfortable discussing cannabis use. That does not mean you should avoid the subject if you have questions about its role in managing your symptoms and optimizing your quality of life.

The National Cancer Institute provides a comprehensive publication on cannabis and cannabinoids. You can access it at https://www.cancer.gov/about-cancer/treatment/cam/patient/cannabis-pdq, or call 1-800-4-CANCER to request a printed copy.

The National Conference of States Legislatures (NCSL) provides the most current information on state laws. Visit www.ncsl.org and type "state medical marijuana laws" in the search bar.

Aches And Pains

Aches and pains can be a side effect of cancer treatment or a symptom of the cancer itself. You will find tips on managing achiness, peripheral neuropathy, and pain below. Knowing how to manage or prevent pain can have a big impact on quality of life.

ACHINESS

Muscle aches are known as *myalgia* and joint pain is known as *arthralgia*. You may experience achiness with chemotherapy, targeted therapy, immunotherapy, hormone therapy, and bone marrow stimulants.

What are the risk factors for myalgia and arthralgia?

- Taxanes (paclitaxel/Taxol or docetaxel/Taxotere) can cause both myalgia and arthralgia within the first few days of treatment. This side effect may last 3-5 days and will recur with each treatment.

- Aromatase inhibitors, used to treat postmenopausal women with estrogen-receptor positive breast cancer, can bring about arthralgia.

- Neupogen and Neulasta are sometimes given the day after chemotherapy to stimulate white blood cell production in the bone marrow. These drugs can cause bone pain, which can be intense, and will last for 3-7 days after injection.

- Fibromyalgia pain can flair during cancer treatment.

Tips for Managing Myalgia and Arthralgia
- Warm baths and warm compresses can be soothing to achy muscles.

- Topical pain-relieving creams, ointments, and patches can provide local pain relief. Look for a product that contains one, or a combination of, the following ingredients:
   - Arnica
   - Capsaicin
   - Eucalyptus
   - Camphor
   - Menthol

- Some people find acupuncture and light massage relaxing, but check with your oncologist before engaging in either of these activities.

- Talk with your oncologist about your myalgia and arthralgia. Your doctor may recommend a non-steroidal anti-inflammatory medication (NSAID), like ibuprofen, or give you a prescription for a pain reliever.

- If you are taking an aromatase inhibitor for breast cancer and notice arthralgia, talk with your oncologist. For some women, arthralgia decreases after a few weeks of taking the medication. But if it persists, your oncologist may switch you to a different aromatase inhibitor. Some women find they tolerate one better than another.

- Exercise and movement can be therapeutic. Take a walk, swim in a pool, or try gentle yoga.

Can myalgia and arthralgia be prevented?

- If your oncologist has suggested a nonsteroidal anti-inflammatory (NSAID), or has given you a prescription pain reliever, try taking the recommended medication the night of treatment and continuing for 2-3 days after. This may help prevent or lessen the severity of myalgia and arthralgia. It is easier to prevent the pain than it is to manage it once it appears.

- If you will be receiving filgrastim (Neupogen or Neulasta) to increase your white blood cell count, ask your oncologist if you can start taking an antihistamine the day of the injection and for a few days after. The antihistamine works by reducing the release of histamines and decreasing inflammation and bone pain.

PERIPHERAL NEUROPATHY

Some chemotherapy drugs can damage the nerves in fingers, hands, toes, and feet, causing a side effect called *peripheral neuropathy*. Peripheral neuropathy can be experienced at any time during your cancer treatment and may increase with each treatment cycle. For some it may be a nuisance. For others it may be physically disabling.

What are the signs and symptoms of peripheral neuropathy?
- Tingling or a pins-and-needles feeling in the fingers and/or toes
- Burning feeling in hands and bottoms of feet
- Sensitivity to touch or temperature
- Decreased sensation or numbness in the fingers, hands, toes, and or feet
- Difficulty picking up small items or buttoning clothes
- Difficulty walking, tripping or stumbling

What are the risk factors for peripheral neuropathy?
- Certain chemotherapy drugs can cause neuropathy.
- Advanced age
- Poor nutrition
- Diabetes or thyroid conditions
- Pre-existing neuropathy

Tips for Managing Peripheral Neuropathy
Some people find that their neuropathy is most pronounced a few days after treatment and lessens just before the next treatment is due. Others may experience worsening of neuropathy with each treatment and may only begin to notice improvement 6-12 months after treatment completion. Symptoms for others remain long-term.
- First and foremost, communicate with your oncologist. Let your oncologist know if you experience any symptoms of peripheral neuropathy. Be specific in describing the pain, frequency, and how it is affecting your ability to function.

- Your oncologist may alter the treatment schedule or frequency to give you some relief and prevent worsening of symptoms.
- Prescription pain relievers, antidepressants, and antiseizure medications can help with pain management.
- A referral to a physical or occupational therapist may be helpful.
- A neurologist may be able to assess the extent of nerve damage and help you manage the pain.

- Protect your hands from injury.
  - Wear gloves when doing housework or yardwork.
  - Avoid exposure to very hot water.
  - Use a kitchen mitt to avoid burns when cooking.

- Protect your feet from injury.
  - Avoid going barefoot. Wear comfortable shoes with good support and good traction. Wear non-slip socks or slippers when indoors.
  - Order diabetic socks online or through a pharmacy. These socks are typically seamless and non-elastic in order to reduce pressure and prevent blisters.
  - Avoid very hot showers or baths.
  - Inspect your feet daily. Clean any open areas or blisters with soap and water, then pat dry. Apply antibacterial ointment and a bandage to prevent infection.

- If you are diabetic, follow up with your endocrinologist or primary physician so your blood sugars are well-managed.

- Practice safety when walking. Make certain you keep a night light on in case you must get up at night. Avoid walking on uneven surfaces to avoid stumbling.

- Acupuncture, massage, and guided imagery may facilitate comfort.

Can peripheral neuropathy be prevented?

- If you are receiving a chemotherapy drug that may cause neuropathy, you can try cold therapy to prevent or reduce the intensity of peripheral neuropathy. Cold therapy involves placing fingers in an ice water bath and feet on cold packs while being infused with the neuropathy-causing drug.

- Vitamin B6 and glutamine powder are two supplements that have been found to reduce the effects of neuropathy in chemotherapy patients. Talk with your oncologist before trying any supplement.

PAIN

Although many people with cancer will have pain at one point or another, having cancer does not guarantee you will have pain. For those who do experience pain, it can have a huge impact on quality of life. Pain affects appetite, interferes with sleep, and makes enjoying physical and social activities difficult. Pain is one of the most feared side effects and can be emotionally frustrating and depressing.

Cancer pain is not something that should be accepted as inevitable. It should not be accepted as your burden to bare. Cancer pain can be controlled and it is your right to have your pain addressed. The first step is to talk with your cancer treatment team and your loved ones and describe what you are experiencing. Your pain is yours alone and no two people experience pain in quite the same way.

We discussed myalgia/arthralgia and peripheral neuropathy above. Other types of pain occur with cancer and cancer treatment. *Acute pain* occurs suddenly and lasts for a short period of time. It can range from mild to severe. *Chronic pain* is pain that has been present for more than 3 months. *Breakthrough pain* is an exacerbation of pain that occurs while taking pain medication.

What are the risk factors for developing pain?

- Surgery

- Chemotherapy or radiation therapy

- Having a tumor that is pressing on an organ or nerve

- Having a tumor involving the bone

- Having a tumor that blocks or obstructs the function of an organ

Tips for Managing Cancer Pain

- The first step in managing cancer pain is talking with your cancer treatment team. It helps to keep a pain diary so you can give a detailed picture of the extent of your pain. Make sure to include the following:
  - How would you rate your pain on a scale of 1-10, with 10 being the worst and 1 being the least pain? If you are not able to give it a number, would you describe it as mild, moderate, or severe?
  - Where is your pain?

- What does it feel like? Is it sharp, shooting, dull, achy, throbbing, or burning?
- When does the pain occur?
- What makes it better? What makes it worse?

• Ask for detailed instructions to help you manage your pain.

• In your pain diary, note the date and time, level of pain, and what you did to relieve the pain. Keep track of when you take pain medications.

• Short-acting pain medication is best used for acute pain.
  - Controlling acute pain is easier when it begins, so take your medication at the first sign of pain.
  - If you find you need your pain medication around the clock, or you are having difficulty waiting for the next scheduled dose, notify the prescribing physician so medication can be adjusted.

• Long-acting and extended-release pain medication is meant to keep pain under control over a 24-hour period.
  - It needs to be taken consistently on schedule and is not meant to be used on an as-needed basis.
  - If you find that you have occasional breakthrough pain, inform the prescribing physician as you may benefit from taking a short-acting pain medicine when needed.
  - If you are taking a short-acting medication for breakthrough pain and find that you are needing it more often, inform your ordering physician so pain medication can be adjusted.

- Following are non-pharmaceutical methods of relieving pain:
  - Biofeedback—a non-invasive therapy which teaches patients to control bodily processes that are normally involuntary
  - Breathing exercises
  - Heat or cold
  - Menthol-based or capsaicin-based creams, gels, or lotions
  - Guided imagery
  - Meditation
  - Massage
  - Acupuncture
  - Transcutaneous nerve stimulators (TENS)
  - Exercise
  - Physical therapy or aquatherapy
  - Radiation therapy to help relieve pain from bone metastasis or decrease the size of a tumor that is pressing on a nerve or organ
  - Surgery to relieve tumor pressure or relieve a blockage or obstruction
  - Nerve block

- Many cancer centers and hospitals have palliative care teams that focus on pain and symptom management with the goal of improving quality of life. You may ask your oncologist for a referral.

- Pain management physicians specialize in addressing all types of pain. Your oncologist can make a referral if your pain is not well controlled.

- Keep your entire care team abreast of medications you are taking so your pain can be addressed without an overlap of medications.

- Narcotics and opioids cause constipation. This type of constipation is not relieved with prunes or increased fiber in the diet. If you are taking prescription pain medication, make sure to keep your bowels moving every day. Over-the-counter stool softeners should be used to keep bowels movements soft and regular. Ask your oncologist which stool softener is recommended. If you find that you have difficulty keeping your bowels moving, talk with your oncologist about a bowel regimen. Prescription medications are also available.

Misconceptions About Cancer Pain

- Narcotics and opioid medications should be avoided because they cause addiction.

- Pain medication makes people drowsy and confused.

- Narcotics and opioid medications should be reserved for people whose disease is advanced.

The truth is pain can interfere with sleep, mood, healing, and overall wellbeing. When pain is managed, healing can take place and each day becomes less of a struggle. Addicts take pain medication because they crave the feeling of being high. If you are taking pain medication for the sole purpose of relieving pain, the risk of addiction is very low.

Yes, you may feel drowsy or dizzy when you first start a prescription medication, but your body will adjust after a few days. You may find that you sleep a lot once you start a prescription pain medication. Your body is finally getting relief from fighting pain and may need to catch up on sleep. Sleepiness will decrease over the course of a few days.

As we discussed above, pain can be a result of cancer treatment or the cancer itself. It can happen at any time over the course of treatment and, although it can be an indication of advanced cancer, it does not necessarily mean that the cancer has gotten worse. Every person has the right to comfort and quality of life. You don't have to accept or endure pain.

Blood And Bone Marrow Side Effects

The goal of cancer treatment is to kill cancer cells, but, as discussed previously, it can also damage healthy cells that divide rapidly, including cells in the bone marrow. If you receive radiation therapy that targets areas with long bones—spine, chest, legs, or pelvis—the cells in your bone marrow may be affected. Chemotherapy can also kill cells in your bone marrow. Your bone marrow plays a vital role in producing white blood cells, red blood cells, and platelets. Cancer treatment can affect any or all of these cells.

ANEMIA

Red blood cells (RBC) carry oxygen and iron through your body. The oxygen carrying part of the RBC is called hemoglobin (Hgb). Chemotherapy can affect the cells that produce red blood cells, as can radiation that targets the bone. Some types of cancer also affect the number of red blood cells in the body. Oncologists monitor the red blood cell levels by doing a blood test called a CBC, or complete blood count. This test will show the number of RBCs as well as the amount of Hgb. Anemia occurs when Hgb is low.

What are signs and symptoms of anemia?

- Your oncologist or nurse should be notified if you are experiencing the following signs and symptoms of anemia:
  - Fatigue
  - Shortness of breath when doing normal activities
  - Pale skin, gums, and tongue
  - Dizziness
  - Rapid heart rate

What are the risk factors for developing anemia?

- Having a history of anemia

- Cancer that affects the blood or bone marrow

- Poor nutritional intake

- Chemotherapy that affects the bone marrow

- Radiation that targets the bones

Tips for Managing Anemia

- Pace your activities to conserve energy.

- Take breaks if you begin to feel short of breath.

- Stand up slowly to avoid dizziness.

- Eat a diet that includes proteins, whole grains, fruits, and vegetables.

- Take walks or do gentle yoga to increase your strength and stamina.

- Your oncologist will monitor your RBC and Hgb throughout treatment. If you are symptomatic, and your levels are low, your oncologist may order a blood transfusion.

- Your oncologist may prescribe a medication to help stimulate the production of more red blood cells.

Can anemia be prevented?

Chemotherapy and radiation therapy can damage the cells in the bone marrow, leading to anemia. Although you can do nothing to prevent this, you can strengthen your body and hasten healing by following the tips above.

NEUTROPENIA

Neutrophils are a type of white blood cell (WBC) that play an important role in helping your body fight infection. Chemotherapy and radiation can have an impact on the number of neutrophils in the blood, putting you at risk for infection. Your oncologist will monitor the number of WBCs with a CBC blood test that measures your complete blood count. Your oncologist may also look at the number of neutrophils in your blood to determine whether your body is prepared for treatment.

WBCs are usually at their lowest 7-10 days after chemotherapy administration. This period is referred to as *nadir.* If the absolute neutrophil count (ANC) falls below 1500, it is called *neutropenia.* If you develop neutropenia, your body will not have the number of neutrophils to help fight foreign invaders, putting you at risk of infection.

What are the signs of neutropenia?

- ANC<1500

- Although a fever is not an indication of neutropenia, a fever may be the only sign of infection in someone with neutropenia.

What are the risk factors for developing neutropenia?

- Chemotherapy drugs that are known to affect the bone marrow

- Radiation therapy that targets the bones

- A past history of neutropenia from past or present chemotherapy

- Having a tumor in the bone marrow

Tips for Managing Neutropenia and Avoiding Infection

- If your WBC or ANC is low, chemotherapy treatments may need to be delayed, or doses reduced, to prevent complications.

- Because the risk of infection is high in a person who has neutropenia, always practice infection precautions.
  - Wash your hands often.
  - Take hand sanitizer with you and use it before and after contact with people.
  - Wipe down surfaces of telephones, smart phones, and tablets with alcohol or sanitizer.
  - Use hand sanitizer after touching objects that are used by the public, such as shopping carts.

- Avoid anyone with a suspected infection.
- Avoid crowds. If you must be in a crowded place, such as a store or airport, wear a mask.
- If you must shop, try going at times when the store is least busy.
- Avoid eating at buffets or salad bars, and avoid eating raw fish or sushi.
- Make sure your food is properly cooked.
- If you develop neutropenia, avoid raw fruits and vegetables, unless they can be peeled before eating.

• A fever may be the first and only sign of an infection. If you develop a temperature above 100.5F, inform your oncologist immediately. Neutropenic fevers must be treated with antibiotics right away.

Can neutropenia be prevented?

• No magic-bullet foods can help prevent neutropenia, but your body will heal quicker if it is properly nourished. Lean proteins, fruits, vegetables, and whole grains help build and strengthen the immune system.

• If you are receiving chemotherapy that has the potential to impact your WBC, your oncologist may choose to give you an injection of filgrastim (Neupogen or Neulasta) the day after treatment. Filgrastim stimulates the bone marrow to produce more WBC, lowering your risk of neutropenia.

THROMBOCYTOPENIA

Platelets, or thrombocytes, are a type of blood cell formed in the bone marrow. They are responsible for clotting your blood. When an injury occurs, these cells rush to the area of injury and form a clot. Because chemotherapy can affect the cells in your bone marrow, the number of platelets in your body may decrease. If your platelet count is low, you may be at risk of bruising and bleeding. The risk of bleeding increases as the platelet count decreases. Platelet counts usually recover on their own, but recovery can be slow. If platelet counts are below 150,000/mm^3, it is called *thrombocytopenia*.

What are signs of thrombocytopenia?

- Bruising easily or excessive bruising—*purpura*

- Reddish-purple spots under the skin—*petechiae*

- Bleeding from gums when brushing teeth

- Nose bleeds

- Blood in urine

- Blood in stool

- Excessive or prolonged bleeding from a cut

- Fatigue

What are the risk factors for developing thrombocytopenia?

- Platelet count <15,000/mm^3

- Chemotherapy that affects the bone marrow

- Radiation therapy targeting bone

- Cancer that involves the blood or bone marrow

Tips for Managing Thrombocytopenia

- Use a soft-bristled toothbrush and avoid using dental floss.

- Be gentle when blowing your nose.

- Use an electric razor to shave.

- Avoid taking any medications without your oncologist's approval, as some medications can thin the blood or slow clot formation.

- Avoid dental work until platelet counts recover.

- An over-the-counter stool softener may be necessary to keep your bowels soft and moving.

- Do not use suppositories or enemas until your platelet count recovers.

- Apply pressure for at least 10 minutes after any injections.

- Call your oncologist if you experience any of the following:
  ○ A nosebleed that lasts longer than 10 minutes after applying pressure to the bridge of the nose
  ○ Spontaneous bleeding not caused by an injury
  ○ Blood in your urine or stool

Can thrombocytopenia be prevented?

Chemotherapy and radiation therapy can affect the cells in the bone marrow, causing thrombocytopenia. There are no effective preventive measures you can take. If your platelet count continues to be low between chemotherapy treatments, your oncologist may need to change the frequency or strength of your chemotherapy. Sometimes a transfusion with platelets is necessary to bring the platelet count up. Oprelvekin (Neumega) is an injection that can be used if platelet counts are chronically low.

Co-Existing Conditions Affected By Chemotherapy

DIABETES

It can be especially challenging to manage diabetes while undergoing cancer treatment. Dexamethasone and prednisone are steroids commonly prescribed to help decrease inflammation, prevent chemotherapy side effects, and manage cancer symptoms. Although they can be an important part of cancer treatment, they can cause problems for those who have diabetes. Steroids affect the body's ability to use insulin and increase the production of glucose in the liver. This can lead to elevated blood sugar levels, a condition known as *hyperglycemia*. If you are diabetic your blood sugar levels might increase for a few days after chemotherapy. You may also find that you have an increased risk of peripheral neuropathy.

Another challenge facing those with diabetes and cancer is low blood sugar, known as *hypoglycemia*. Appetite may be affected by cancer treatment. Nausea, vomiting, and diarrhea can lead to dehydration and hypoglycemia.

What are the signs of hyperglycemia?

- Increased thirst
- Increased urination
- Blurry vision
- Tingling in hands and feet

What are the risk factors for developing hyperglycemia?

- History of diabetes

- Being overweight

- Smoking

- Cancer of the pancreas

- Alcohol use

- Inactivity

- Steroid use

- Use of nutritional supplements

- Change in eating habits

What are the signs of hypoglycemia?

- Shakiness or jittery feeling

- Sleepiness

- Dizziness

- Confusion

- Increased heart rate

What are the risk factors for developing hypoglycemia?

- Nausea and vomiting

- Diarrhea

- Decreased appetite

- The use of oral diabetic medications and/or insulin use

Tips for Managing Diabetes During Cancer Treatment

- Do not ignore your diabetes because you are being treated for cancer. Increased blood sugar can stress the immune system, prolong wound healing, damage the kidneys, increase the risk of infection, and negatively impact overall prognosis.

- If you are not being followed by an endocrinologist, ask your oncologist for a referral. Endocrinologists are specially trained to manage diabetes and should be included as part of your cancer care team. They can help develop a medication plan to keep tight control of your blood sugars.

- A sliding scale of insulin may be prescribed, in which your insulin dose is based on your blood sugar levels.

- If you are instructed to check your blood sugars, be consistent. Keep a journal with your blood sugar readings and what you did to manage your blood sugar. Bring this journal with you to your endocrinologist.

- Exercise on a regular basis to help lower blood sugar.

- Proper nutrition is key to managing diabetes, especially during cancer treatment.
  - Ask for a referral to a diabetic educator, nutritionist, or dietitian so you can learn how to optimize nutrition and keep blood sugar levels in balance.
  - Eat on a regular schedule. Keep healthy, portable snacks on hand so you avoid going long periods of time without eating.
  - Avoid sugary drinks and supplements.

○ Increase your intake of healthy fats and whole grains. These foods tend to be filling and help keep your blood sugar at an even level.

○ Increase your intake of vegetables.

○ Decrease your intake of empty calories, such as cookies, cakes, white bread, and potato chips.

HYPERTENSION

Hypertension, also known as high blood pressure, is a common co-existing condition in cancer patients as one out of every three Americans has hypertension. Hypertension occurs when the force of blood through your vessels is too high. Certain cancer treatments can increase blood pressure, either bringing on a new diagnosis of hypertension or exacerbating an existing condition. When blood pressure increases, it puts stress on the walls of the arteries and increases the risk of plaque formation. If untreated, hypertension can lead to cardiac disease, stroke, and kidney failure.

What are the signs of hypertension?

- Systolic pressure >140 and diastolic pressure >90

- Severe headache described as a pounding or pressure in the head

- A sudden rise in blood pressure may cause
  ○ Fatigue and confusion
  ○ Blurry vision
  ○ Chest pain and pressure
  ○ Shortness of breath
  ○ Irregular heartbeat
  ○ Pounding in the chest and/or ears

What are the risk factors for hypertension?

- Family history of hypertension
- Being male over 45 years of age or female over 65 years of age
- Being African American
- Being overweight
- Smoking
- A diet high in fat and salt
- Alcohol
- Lack of exercise or physical activity
- Diabetes
- Kidney disease
- Sleep apnea
- Certain cancer treatments can increase the risk of hypertension or exacerbate existing conditions. Examples include:
  - Pertuzumab (Perjeta)
  - Bevacizumab (Avastin)
  - Sunitinib (Sutent)
  - Sorafenib (Nexavar)
  - Traztuzumab (Herceptin)

Tips for Managing Hypertension

- If you have a history of hypertension, inform your oncologist so you can be monitored closely.
- If you have a history of hypertension, check your blood pressure daily and keep a log of the results. Inform your physician if blood pressure rises above 140/90.

- Increase your intake of fruit, vegetables, lean protein, and whole grains.

- Decrease your intake of fried and processed food.

- Decrease your intake of salt. Make sure to read labels for sodium content.

- Limit sugar intake.

- Exercise every day. Movement increases blood flow and strengthens the cardiovascular system. It also increases energy and helps fight fatigue.

- If you smoke, talk to your physician about options to help you quit.

- Limit alcohol intake.

- Practice stress management and mindfulness techniques.

- Schedule regular follow ups with a family physician or cardiologist who can oversee the treatment of your blood pressure.

- Medications may be necessary to keep your blood pressure at a healthy level.

Eye Issues

Chemotherapy, steroids, targeted therapy, and hormone therapy can cause eye problems and changes in vision. Steroids can cause blurry vision. This will improve once steroids are no longer being used. Tamoxifen increases the risk of cataracts. Some chemotherapy drugs affect the tear ducts and can cause irritation and excessive tearing.

What are the signs and symptoms of treatment-related eye issues?

- Blurry vision

- Dry eyes

- Watery, teary eyes

- Light sensitivity

- Redness and irritation

What are risk factors for developing eye issues?

- Some types of chemotherapy

- Hormone therapy

- Steroids

Tips for Managing Eye Issues

- Artificial tears work well to manage dry eyes.

- You can use baby shampoo and warm water to clean your eyelids.

- If you notice that your eyes are irritated, red, and/or excessively teary, inform your oncologist for further evaluation.

Can eye issues be prevented?

- If possible, schedule an eye exam before starting treatment.

- Avoid wearing contacts during cancer treatment, as they may irritate your eyes and can be a source of infection.

- Inform your oncologist of any eye-related issues before starting treatment.

Fatigue And Sleep

Fatigue is one of the most pervasive side effects of cancer and its treatments. It is more than being tired. When you are tired, a good night's sleep or a nap can leave you feeling refreshed. Not so with fatigue. With fatigue, you never quite feel fully alert and energized, which may be difficult for family and friends to understand.

Fatigue can be caused by the cancer itself. Cancer cells stimulate the release of cytokines, protein messengers that are part of the immune system. Cytokines initiate an inflammatory response in the body and this causes fatigue. Cancer cells also require nutrients to grow, leaving less for the body to use.

Cancer treatments can further zap energy. The body needs to muster all its energy sources to repair itself after surgery. Surgery is usually followed by chemotherapy or radiation, giving little time to recover. Fatigue usually occurs within a few days of receiving chemotherapy. It may increase a bit the week before the next session, but decrease with each subsequent treatment. With radiation therapy, fatigue may begin around the third or fourth week and may increase as treatment progresses.

Imagine the body as a boxer fighting in a ring. With the first cancer treatment, the boxer stumbles and gets back up. With the next punch of treatment, the boxer staggers and takes a bit longer to get up. As the boxer continues to fight, energy decreases. It may take a while to recover that energy. Anemia, neutropenia, and thrombocytopenia can add to fatigue, as can the medications prescribed to relieve cancer symptoms and treatment side effects. Many people are surprised to find that fatigue can last long after cancer treatment is finished.

What are the signs of fatigue?

- Groggy after a full night sleep

- Difficulty getting up in the morning

- An overwhelming feeling of being tired

- Difficulty concentrating

- Shortness of breath after normal activity

- Sudden feeling of exhaustion

- Lack of motivation

- Decreased endurance

- Feeling weak

- Feeling sad, depressed, or irritable

What are risk factors for fatigue?

- Receiving combination of cancer treatments

- Anemia, neutropenia, and/or thrombocytopenia

- Pain

- Depression

- Advanced cancer

- A history of heart problems

- Obesity

- Diabetes

- Nausea, vomiting, diarrhea

- Medications for pain

- Medications for nausea and vomiting

- Antidepressants

- Poor nutrition

- Lack of exercise

Tips for Managing Fatigue

- Try to go to sleep and wake up at the same time every day.

- Naps can be rejuvenating. Naps are best before 3 p.m. Avoid napping longer than an hour so as not to disrupt your body's sleep-wake cycle.

- Prioritize activities. If you would like to do something, plan to rest before and after so you can enjoy the activity.

- Pace yourself. Break activities and tasks into short periods with rest time in between.

- Set boundaries. Accept help from others. Ask for help when needed. And say *no* if you need to rest.

- Stay hydrated. Dehydration can put stress on the body, adding to fatigue.

- Talk with your oncologist about your fatigue and any unmanaged symptoms or side effects. Pain, nausea, diarrhea, and poor appetite contribute to energy loss. Some medications cause drowsiness. Your oncologist can help manage these side effects and may be able to change medications to lessen drowsiness.

- Depression can contribute to lack of motivation and fatigue. Support groups, counseling, and meditation can be helpful.

Ask your physician for resources to help manage your emotions.

Can fatigue be prevented?

Fatigue is an inherent side effect of cancer treatment. You may not be able to prevent fatigue, but you can lessen its impact. Whole food nutrition and exercise are paramount.

- **Nutrition**
  - Small frequent meals may be easier to digest than three big meals.
  - Include protein in every meal. Lean sources of protein include beans, nut butters, chicken, fish, quinoa, yogurt, and cottage cheese.
  - Vegetables and fruits add powerful nutrients that help repair cells and boost the immune system.
  - Keep your pantry and refrigerator stocked with foods that are quick and easy to prepare.
  - See Chapter 6 for more information on nutrition.
  - See the Appendix B for recipes.

- **Exercise**
  - Although pacing and scheduling rest time is wise to do when you are fatigued, the importance of exercise cannot be stressed enough. There will be days when it takes a lot of motivation and effort to get out of the chair and exercise, but your body will be better for it.
  - Exercise has several benefits:
    - Helps increase muscle mass and flexibility
    - Helps control weight, which decreases the risk of cancer recurrence

- Improves blood flow and decreases the risk of developing clots in the legs
- Strengthens the bones, decreasing the risk of osteoporosis
- Improves balance, decreasing the risk of falls
- Releases endorphins, improving mood and decreasing depression
- Improves lung function
- Increases appetite and aids in digestion
- Increases endurance and is one of the best ways to decrease fatigue

○ Schedule exercise into your day and make it a priority. Try to exercise when you seem to have the most energy.

○ The goal is 30 minutes of activity at least 5 days a week. If 30 minutes seems beyond your reach, try spreading it throughout the day by doing 5-10 minutes of activity at a time.

○ If you were active prior to your diagnosis, you may find that you need to change goals and expectations.

○ If you were sedentary when treatment started, set small goals and start slowly. The important thing is that you do some type of activity on a regular basis.

○ If standing is difficult, try chair exercises. You can use soup cans or water bottles as weights to work your arm muscles. You can do leg raises while seated or hold onto a chair and march in place.

○ Resistance bands come in a variety of strengths to suit beginner to athlete. They can be used sitting or standing and provide a safe way to work muscles and increase flexibility.

○ Many cancer centers offer exercise classes for cancer patients.

○ Yoga and tai chi benefit the mind and body by increasing flexibility and inducing relaxation.

○ Try walking, dancing, or gardening.

○ If you need motivation, enlist a buddy to exercise with you.

○ Make sure to stay hydrated, wear sunblock and a hat when outdoors, and avoid exercising outside during the heat of the day.

SLEEP DISTURBANCES

Sleep is essential for a healthy mind and body. A good night's sleep helps regulate blood sugar, power up the immune system, and enhance memory. It is estimated that about 50 percent of cancer patients have difficulty getting a good night's sleep. Without a full night's sleep of 7-8 hours, the immune system is stressed.

What are signs of sleep disturbance?

• Insomnia—difficulty falling asleep

• Difficulty staying asleep

• Waking early with inability to fall back to sleep

What are risk factors for sleep disturbances?

• Stress

• Treatment side effects

- Pain

- Steroid medications

- Hot flashes

- Alcohol use

Tips for Managing Sleep Disturbances

- Try to establish a regular sleep-wake cycle by going to sleep and rising at the same time every day.

- Develop a bedtime ritual that tells your brain it is time to slow down and settle for bed.

- If you are not able to fall asleep, do not fight it. Try going in another room. Read. Listen to music.

- Limit naps to 30 minutes at a time. Do not nap after 3 p.m. to avoid difficulty falling asleep later.

- Use the bed only for sleep or intimacy. Avoid eating or watching TV in bed. This will help your body associate the bed with sleep.

- Avoid caffeine or alcohol at least 4 hours before bed.

- A warm bath, a cup of chamomile tea, and a light snack can be helpful.

- Try listening to ambient noise, available on some alarm clocks and smart phone apps.

- Guided imagery, deep breathing, and meditation can help clear the mind, decrease anxiety, and prepare you for sleep.

- Address underlying causes of sleep disturbances:

- If nausea, diarrhea, or pain is interfering with sleep, speak with your oncologist or nurse about adjusting your medications or the times you take them to help you sleep through the night.
- Hot flashes can interfere with sleep. Try wearing cotton pajamas, keeping a fan by your bed, and using a cool gel pillow. Your oncologist may also prescribe a medication to help decrease the intensity and frequency of hot flashes.

Fluid Retention

EDEMA

Edema is an abnormal build-up of fluid under the skin. It occurs most commonly in the hands, arms, feet, and legs.

What are the signs of edema?

- Swelling of fingers, hands, arms, feet, and or legs

- Clothes, rings or shoes feel tight

- Indentation of the skin when pressed

- Skin feels tight and looks shiny

- Sudden weight gain

- Decreased flexibility of the extremity

- Puffy, full, heavy feeling in the extremity

What are the risk factors for edema?

- Some types of chemotherapy cause fluid retention, such as cisplatin (Platinol) and docetaxol (Taxotere).

- Steroids

- Inactivity

- Low levels of protein

- Blood clots

- Hormone therapy

- Problems with kidney, liver, or heart function

Tips for Managing Edema

- Decrease your salt intake.

- Elevate the swollen extremity. You can prop feet up on a table or stool when seated. Use pillows at night to make sure the swollen extremity is above the level of your heart.

- Avoid crossing your legs.

- Avoid tight shoes.

- Compression hose can help decrease edema in the legs and feet.

- Discuss fluid retention and edema with your oncologist. Sometimes medications can be changed to decrease the risk of edema. Diuretics may be ordered to help rid excess fluid.

- Call your oncologist if you notice the following:
  - Sudden shortness of breath and racing heart
  - Sudden swelling
  - Swelling that occurs in only one extremity and only on one side
  - Pain when using the affected extremity
  - Redness and/or heat in the affected extremity
  - Sudden weight gain
  - Decreased or difficulty urinating

Can edema be prevented?

Although some chemotherapy and medications can cause fluid retention, you can take steps to decrease your risk.

- Focus on drinking at least ten 8-ounce glasses of fluids each day. It may sound counterintuitive to increase fluids when you are trying to avoid fluid retention, but fluids help keep kidneys working and help flush waste from the body.

- Make sure you nourish your body with protein, fruits, and vegetables.

- Avoid sitting or standing for long periods of time. Fluid tends to pool when you remain in one position for too long. This increases the risk of blood clots.

LYMPHEDEMA

Lymphedema is the buildup of lymph fluid in fatty tissue beneath the skin. Lymph fluid contains protein, salts, water, and infection-fighting white blood cells. This fluid flows through a network of vessels called the lymphatic system. As lymph fluid travels, it passes through lymph nodes, which act as filters to pick up debris and destroy germs. When lymph nodes are damaged or removed, the flow of lymph fluid is impeded. The fluid may build up and cause swelling—lymphedema.

What are signs of lymphedema?

- Swelling
  - If lymph nodes were removed in the axilla, you may note swelling of the chest, underarm, arm, and hand.

- If lymph nodes were removed from the pelvic area or groin, or you have had radiation therapy to this area, you may experience swelling of the genitals or leg.
- Radiation therapy, or removal of lymph nodes in the neck area, can result in swelling of the face and neck.

- Tight feeling clothes, rings, watches, or shoes

- A heavy sensation in the affected extremity

- Achiness in the affected extremity

- Tightness of the skin

- Decreased range of motion

What are the risk factors for lymphedema?

- Lymph node removal—lymph node dissection

- Radiation therapy of the neck, groin, axilla, pelvis

Tips for Managing Lymphedema

- Report signs and symptoms of lymphedema to your physician as soon as you note them.

- Ask for a referral to a certified lymphedema therapist (CLT). A CLT has received training in treating and preventing lymphedema.
  - A CLT will treat lymphedema with a technique called manual lymphatic drainage. The area of lymphedema will be gently massaged so that lymph fluid will drain properly and swelling will be reduced. The CLT will teach you or a loved one how to do manual lymphatic drainage at home.

○ You may be fitted for a compression sleeve or stocking to help put constant pressure on the affected area, thereby decreasing swelling.

○ Complete Decompressive Therapy (CDT) is the most comprehensive way of treating and managing lymphedema. The goal is to treat existing lymphedema and teach techniques to prevent it from occurring in the future. The therapy consists of manual lymphatic drainage, the use of compression garments, exercises, skin care, and education in self-management.

• Exercise may help increase the flow of lymph fluid. A physical therapist or CLT can show you appropriate exercises.

• Skin care is imperative because lymphedema increases the risk of infection.
  ○ Keep the affected area clean and moisturized.
  ○ Avoid injury to the affected area.
  ○ Keep antibacterial ointment with you at all times. If you do receive a cut or burn to the area, clean with soap and water and apply the ointment right away.
  ○ Protect the area from sun exposure. Use a sunscreen with SPF of at least 30.

• Cellulitis is an infection under the skin in the affected extremity. It is a serious complication of lymphedema, as infection can quickly spread throughout the extremity and the body. If you have lymphedema, be aware of the signs and symptoms of cellulitis and report them to your physician immediately. Signs and symptoms include:

- ◦ Redness, heat, and tenderness in the affected extremity
- ◦ A streaky red line or splotchy redness in the affected extremity
- ◦ Fever and chills
- ◦ Pain

Can lymphedema be prevented?

When lymph nodes are damaged or removed, they do not grow back. If you have had a lymph node dissection, or radiation therapy to lymph nodes, you will be always be at risk of lymphedema. Ask for a referral to a CLT once you have healed from surgery. A CLT can teach you techniques to prevent and self-manage lymphedema. You can also follow the tips below:

- Keep your skin clean and use moisturizer daily.

- Avoid compression to the extremity. Do not allow blood pressure or needle sticks in the affected extremity. Avoid carrying bags or purses with the strap on the affected arm.

- Avoid constricting clothes or jewelry.

- Avoid cuts or bruises. Keep antibacterial hand sanitizer and antibiotic ointment on hand to clean any open areas.

- Avoid extremely hot showers, baths, and hot tubs.

- Keep nails clean and trim but avoid cutting cuticles.

- Wear gloves when doing housework or gardening.

- Use a sunscreen with a minimum of SPF 30.

- Use insect repellant when appropriate to avoid bites, which can lead to infection.

- Maintain a healthy weight, as being overweight increases the risk of lymphedema.

- Exercise is an essential part of preventing lymphedema. Exercise should be gradual and decreased or stopped if pain or swelling is noted. Stretching exercises, weight bearing exercises, and aerobic activity is recommended. A personal trainer experienced in working with cancer patients can be helpful in developing a program that is right for you.

Hair

ALOPECIA

Hair loss, or *alopecia,* can be one of the most distressing side effects of cancer treatment. Because chemotherapy kills cells that divide most rapidly, it can affect skin, hair, and nails. Not all chemotherapy causes hair loss. Your chemotherapy nurse will let you know if you can expect hair loss with your treatment. Radiation therapy can also cause hair loss, but only in the area being radiated.

What are signs of alopecia?

- You may notice an achiness, itchiness, or tingling sensation on your scalp just before your hair begins to fall out.

- Hair loss can occur slowly or rapidly. Some people notice a thinning of their hair, while others lose all of the hair, including eyelashes, eyebrows, and pubic hair.

- Hair loss usually begins 2-4 weeks after starting treatment.

- You may notice hair on your pillowcase, in the shower, or on your comb or brush.

- Some people lose only the hair on their head. Others may lose eyebrows, eyelashes, body hair, armpit hair, and pubic hair.

- If you are receiving radiation therapy, you may notice hair loss in the area that is being radiated.

- You can expect your hair to begin growing back within 3-6 months of completing chemotherapy. Your new hair may be a different color or texture when it comes back.

What are risk factors for alopecia?

- Some chemotherapy drugs can cause hair loss.

- Radiation therapy can cause hair loss in the area being radiated.

Tips for Managing Alopecia

- Hair loss can be difficult because it affects self-image. Preparing ahead is helpful. Most people find it easier to manage hair loss when their hair is cut short.

- Use a gentle shampoo and avoid using dryers or straighteners.

- Avoid coloring hair until your treatment is complete.

- Purchase a satin pillowcase which is gentle on the hair.

- Use a sunscreen with a minimum SPF of 30 on your scalp if you will be outside without a head covering.

- Turbans, scarves, and hats can be a stylish and comfortable way to cover your head.

- The American Cancer Society offers a free group workshop called Look Good Feel Better. Cosmetologists provide lessons in skin care and nail care. Attendees learn how to style scarves, wigs, and turbans. Each attendee receives an instruction booklet and their own personal bag of cosmetic and skin care products. You can visit the website at www.lookgoodfeelbetter.org or call 1-800-395-5665.

- Wigs come in a variety of colors and styles.
  - Call your insurance company and ask if they provide benefits for a wig. If your insurance company offers wig coverage, you will need a prescription from your oncologist that states "hair prosthesis" before making your purchase.
  - Wigs are made from different materials. Although natural hair wigs may look closer to your own hair, they tend to be expensive. Synthetic wigs are much easier to care for and less expensive.
  - The best way to choose a wig is to try it on. Many wig stores specialize in working with cancer patients and may allow you to schedule a private fitting. You will want to choose a wig before you lose all of your hair and have it resized later.
  - The American Cancer Society offers wigs through their tlc catalogue. You can visit the website at www.tlcdirect.org. You can also order a catalogue by calling 1-800-850-9445.
  - The American Cancer Society offers a wig bank with free wigs to choose from. Call 1-800-227-2345 or visit www.cancer.org to find an office close to you.

Can alopecia be prevented?

Cold cap therapy, or scalp hypothermia, involves the use of a cap that is chilled to a very low temperature and worn throughout chemotherapy infusion. The cold temperature constricts blood vessels, decreasing the blood flow to the scalp, thereby lowering the effects of chemotherapy on the hair follicles and decreasing hair loss. Some health care professionals do not advocate the use of cold caps due to the very small risk of cancer spreading to the scalp. Since this is a rare occurrence, the FDA, at the time of this writing, has approved the DigniCap system for use in cancer treatment centers.

The cold cap must be worn before, during, and after the chemotherapy infusion. Many women report feeling cold and having a headache while wearing the cap. Results vary, with some women having no hair loss and others having significant thinning.

Occasionally, an insurance company will provide some coverage, but the bulk of the expense rests with the patient. The Rapunzel Project is an organization dedicated to providing information about cold cap therapy. You can visit their site at www.rapunzelproject.org. Hair to Stay is an organization that provides financial support to patients who can't afford cold cap therapy. Their website is www.hairtostay.org.

Memory And Cognition

Up to 75 percent of people undergoing cancer treatment report difficulty with cognitive skills, memory, and focus. You may have heard of chemobrain, but this term is misleading, as cognitive changes can affect any cancer patient, even those not receiving chemotherapy. These changes usually improve over time, but up to 30 percent of cancer patients still experience issues years after cancer treatment has been complete. Studies are being done to better understand this condition.

What are signs of memory and cognitive issues?

- Difficulty focusing, paying attention, concentrating
- Feeling mentally foggy, sometimes termed *brainfog*
- Difficulty recalling names, dates, and phone numbers
- Inability to multitask or stay organized
- Difficulty with math
- Slower thought processes

What are risk factors for memory issues and cognitive changes?

- Chemotherapy or immunotherapy
- Medications used to treat nausea, depression, anxiety, insomnia, and pain
- Hormone therapy
- Radiation therapy
- Stress and anxiety
- Depression
- Brain surgery
- Cancer that has spread to the brain

Tips for Managing Cognitive Changes

- Mark important dates in a calendar, planner, or on your smart phone.
- Store important numbers in your phone and post them in a prominent location in your house.

- Use your smart phone to take pictures of your medication list.

- Use a pill dispenser for daily medications.

- Carry a notepad to jot down information that you want to remember.

- Use sticky notes as reminders.

- Assign a single drop-off spot in the house for important items such as keys, wallet, and phone.

- Have a folder or ringed-binder to keep important papers.

- Keep a list of daily tasks and focus on completing only one at a time.

- Physical activity like walking, gardening, biking, or yoga, has been found to boost cognition and memory.

- Exercise your mind. Word searches, crosswords, math puzzles, and mental challenges can help strengthen brain function. Other activities that can help are playing an instrument, studying a new language, or getting involved in a hobby.

- Meditation can be helpful to clear the mind and enhance memory and recall.

- If you are feeling anxious, stressed, or depressed, discuss this with your physician, as these feelings can impair your ability to think clearly.

- Ask your oncologist for a referral to a speech-language pathologist who does cognitive therapy.

Can cognitive changes be prevented?

Researchers do not yet understand how cancer treatments affect cognitive skills, and there is no way to know who will be affected. The tips above will help strengthen your memory and cognition while undergoing cancer treatment.

Nails

Chemotherapy attacks cells that multiply rapidly, including the fast-growing cells that make up your fingernails and toenails. These changes are temporary and nails will grow out and heal about 6 months after chemotherapy completion.

What are signs of nail changes?

- Darkening of the nails

- White lines across the nail

- Indentations in the nail

- Nail splitting

- Lifting of the nails from the nail bed

- Nail loss

- Dry, cracked cuticles

What are risk factors for developing nail changes?

- The following chemotherapy drugs can cause changes to the fingernails and toenails:
  - Paclitaxel (Taxol)
  - Docetaxol (Taxotere)
  - Fluorouracil (5FU)

- ○ Capecitabine (Xeloda)

- ○ Pegylated doxorubicin (Doxil)

- Diabetes

- Peripheral neuropathy

- Peripheral vascular disease

Tips for Managing Nail Changes

- Keep nails trimmed and clean.

- Use gloves when doing housework, working in the garden, or doing outdoor projects.

- Avoid the use of gel or acrylic nails while undergoing chemotherapy, as these can increase the risk of infection.

- Keep your hands, feet, fingernails and toenails moisturized by using a thick lotion every day. Moisturize your cuticles, too.

- Avoid exposing hands and feet to hot water.

- If you notice your nails lifting, massage them with tea tree oil which acts as a natural anti-fungal. Wrap the nails in bandages to avoid catching them on something.

Can nail changes be prevented?

Nail changes may be difficult to prevent. If you are receiving a taxane (paclitaxel/Taxol or docetaxel/Taxotere), you can try cold therapy. This involves soaking the nails in an ice water bath during the taxane infusion. This slows the blood flow to the nails and decreases the risk of nail changes.

Skin

Skin is the biggest organ of the body and the first line of defense against injury and foreign invaders. It is also one of the most common sites to be affected by cancer treatments. The type of skin reaction you experience will depend on the type of treatment you receive.

ACNEIFORM RASH

Certain drugs used to treat cancer, called epidermal growth factor (EGFR) inhibitors, can affect the epidermal skin cells and cause an acne-like rash. About 90 percent of people receiving EGFR inhibitors will develop a rash. Although it unpleasant and uncomfortable, it is not an allergic reaction. Studies have shown that the rash indicates response to the treatment.

What are signs and symptoms of an acneiform rash?

- The rash may appear on the face, scalp, neck, chest, and back.

- It may appear as red bumps and can be filled with pus. Some people describe it as looking like a bad case of teenage acne.

- It may be itchy, tender, burn or sting.

What are risk factors for developing an acneiform rash?

- Epidermal growth factor (EGFR) inhibitors, including:
  - Cetuximab (Erbitux)
  - Erlotinib (Tarceva)
  - Gefitinib (Iressa)
  - Lapatinib (Tykerb)
  - Panitumumab (Vectibix)

149

Tips for Managing an Acneiform Rash

- Do not use an acne cream to treat the rash.

- Do inform your oncologist. You will be able to continue with treatment, but your oncologist may want to prescribe an antibiotic pill or cream to lessen symptoms.

- Use fragrance-free, mild soap to wash your face.

- Hydrocortisone cream 1% and oatmeal-based lotions may be soothing.

- Always wear PABA-free sunscreen with an SPF of at least 30 when outdoors.

- Avoid hot showers and baths.

- Wear gloves when doing dishes, housework, or working in a garden.

Can an acneiform rash be prevented?

EGFR promotes the growth of hair, skin, and nails. It can also promote the growth of cancer cells. EGFR inhibitors block the growth of cancer cells and can also affect the skin. The acneiform rash is a sign of the body's response to treatment and the rash can't be prevented. If you are receiving an EGFR inhibitor and develop an acneiform rash, inform your oncologist and follow the management tips above.

DRY SKIN

Dryness is one of the most common skin changes noted with cancer treatment.

What are signs and symptoms of dry skin?

- Rough, flaky skin

- Redness and itchiness

- Cracks in the heels of the feet

What are risk factors for dry skin?

- Chemotherapy or immunotherapy

- Radiation therapy

- Dehydration

- Poor nutrition

Tips for Managing Dry Skin

- Use a mild soap, free of perfumes and dyes. Lukewarm water is best for bathing and showering.

- Use sunscreen with a minimum SPF of 30 whenever you will be outdoors. It may be surprising to learn that you can get a sunburn while riding in the car, so make sure that you slather on sunscreen before traveling.

- Increase your intake of fruits, vegetables, healthy fats, and fluids so your skin stays well-hydrated and heals quickly.

- Start your day by applying a thick lotion to your hands and feet.

- Apply a thick lotion before bed, then put on a pair of socks and gloves to help seal in the moisture.

- Avoid using scrubs, loofahs, or chemicals on your skin.

- Coconut oil, shea butter, almond oil, and vitamin E oils are super-hydrating and can be used on face and body.

Can dry skin be prevented?

You can help prevent dry skin by following the tips above.

HAND-FOOT SYNDROME

Some drugs, most notably capecitabine (Xeloda) and liposomal doxorubicin (Doxil), cause a type of hand-foot syndrome known as palmar-plantar erythrodysesthesia (PPE). Targeted therapies can cause PPE, as well.

What are signs and symptoms of hand-foot syndrome?

- The palms and soles of the feet can become red, tender, cracked and blistered.

- Skin may feel tight and burn.

Tips for Managing Hand-Foot Syndrome

If you notice changes in your skin while on cancer treatment, inform your oncologist as soon as you can. A break from treatment or change in your chemotherapy dose may be necessary. If hand-foot syndrome is not addressed when it occurs, it can progress and become painful.

Can hand-foot syndrome be prevented?

If you are receiving Xeloda or Doxil, prevention is the best medicine.

- Avoid placing hands and feet in hot water for an extended period of time. Tepid water is best for baths, showers, and washing hands.

- Try cold therapy. Place feet on ice packs and fingers in ice water during the treatment infusion or, if taking oral chemotherapy, for 15 minute intervals throughout the day.

- Use gloves for outdoor chores, gardening, and housecleaning.

- Keep hands and feet moisturized by using a thick emollient lotion morning and night. Socks and gloves can be worn to bed to keep moisture in.

- Wear socks or slippers in the house. Avoid going barefoot. Choose shoes that are comfortable and don't constrict or pinch your feet.

- Ask your oncologist or nurse if you can take vitamin B6, as it can help prevent hand-foot syndrome.

RADIATION DERMATITIS AND BURNS

Radiation therapy can cause dryness, redness, inflammation, and blistering in the area being radiated. Redness usually begins during the third week of treatment and may increase in intensity as treatment progresses. Because radiation therapy continues to exert its effects for a few weeks after treatment, redness and burning may increase during the last week of treatment and continue for a couple weeks after treatment completion. People who are fair-skinned tend to experience more redness and burning with radiation therapy.

What are the signs and symptoms of radiation burns and dermatitis?

- Redness in the area of radiation therapy

- Redness in the area posterior to the radiation therapy, such as redness of the back when the chest is being irradiated

- Dry, itchy skin in the area of radiation

- Darkening of the irradiated skin

- Burning or tingling sensation

- Pain

- Blistering

- Peeling of the skin

What are the risk factors for radiation-related skin changes?

- Anyone receiving radiation is at risk, but there is a higher risk for fair-skinned individuals

- Poor nutrition

- Diabetes

- History of smoking or alcohol use

- Obesity

- Radiation directed to the head and neck, face, axilla (underarm), rectum, vagina, or skin folds

Tips for Managing Radiation Dermatitis and Burns

- Start caring for your skin from day one of radiation therapy. Apply a cream or emollient to your skin after every radiation treatment and reapply before bed. Do not apply before radiation therapy, as your skin needs to be free of any barriers during treatment.

- You may use aloe vera gel, lanolin cream, 41% petrolatum ointment, shea butter, or coconut oil. Your radiation oncologist may recommend a particular skin cream to use during treatment.

- Keep the area clean and dry. Use a mild, fragrance-free soap to bathe and gently pat the area to dry. You may also use a blow dryer on the cool setting to dry the area.

- Avoid sun exposure to the radiated area. If you must be outside or travel in a car for any length of time, keep the irradiated skin covered and slather sunscreen of SPF 30 or higher on any exposed areas. Consider sun-protective clothing designed with UVA/UVB protection.

- Inform your radiation oncologist if your skin becomes painful or blisters. Hydrogel sheets or honey-based skin sheets can help heal the skin. Your radiation oncologist may also give you a prescription for silver sulfadiazine, a thick white ointment that helps heal burns.

- If you are receiving radiation to the head and neck area, your esophagus may become burned, making it difficult to swallow. Communicate often with your radiation oncologist who can prescribe medications for pain. Your radiation oncologist may suggest the placement of a feeding tube in your belly. This may sound distressing, but it can help rest your esophagus and allow you to get needed nutrition while undergoing treatment. The tube is removed once treatment is complete, the throat has time to heal, and you are able to maintain your weight.

- Radiation to the rectal area or vaginal area can be painful due to skin irritation and burning. The following tips may be helpful:

- Apply one of the skin creams mentioned, or one recommended by your radiation oncologist, after every treatment and before bed.
- Use moistened, alcohol-free, wipes to keep the area clean.
- A sitz bath can be very helpful to sooth irritation and burning.
- Try filling a squeeze bottle with warm water and use it while urinating to decrease irritation.
- Use a cool blow dryer to keep the area dry.
- Talk with your radiation oncologist about any pain you are experiencing so it can be remedied as soon as possible. Your radiation oncologist may also decide to give you a short break from treatment to allow time to heal.

Can radiation-related skin changes be prevented?

You are at risk of skin changes simply by receiving radiation therapy. Although skin changes cannot be prevented, the severity of skin changes can be lessened by using an emollient cream to the irradiated area from day one of treatment, keeping the area clean and dry, and maintaining good nutrition throughout treatment.

The Key To Managing Side Effects

Remember that every person experiences cancer and cancer treatment differently. Talk with your oncology nurse about what side effects are expected with your treatment plan. Ask for written instructions to help prevent and manage side effects so you can be prepared and proactive. Ask questions. Accept support. Take good care of yourself. And take one day at a time.

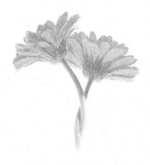

Part IV

Addressing
Difficult Issues

Chapter 9

Sexuality and Intimacy

Sexuality is about how we express ourselves as a person, the clothes we wear, the way we act, how we love, and who we love. It's more about who we are and how we see ourselves than about the physical act of sex. Sexuality helps to define us.

Intimacy, on the other hand, is an affectionate relationship with another person. It's about being physically and emotionally close to someone. Although it can be expressed through sexual activity, intimacy is not about sex. It requires mutual care and concern and a true appreciation for one another. Intimacy is conveyed by talking, listening, physical affection, and sharing experiences together. It makes us feel loved.

Sexuality and intimacy are not topics that often come up in conversation when you are dealing with cancer because the focus is on thriving and surviving. Physicians and nurses tend to avoid the issue when discussing cancer treatment and side effects. But intimacy is an important component of quality of life. It makes a person feel valued, loved, and secure.

Intimacy and affection can be a challenge with all the obstacles cancer throws at you. Intense emotions and physical changes can affect desire and self-esteem. Practical issues, such as family, relationships, finances, and employment, can cause stress and strain on relationships. It may be all too overwhelming to try and relax enough to even think about sexual intimacy.

Your body may look and feel different. It may function differently. You may feel anxious about being intimate with your partner because you feel less attractive. Some people describe feeling broken, physically and emotionally.

Your partner may have anxieties as well. He or she may feel helpless and unsure of how to show affection. Roles and relationships can change throughout the cancer journey, and your partner may be taking on more of a caregiver role.

Intimacy may be the last thing on your mind, but talking about sexuality and intimacy is important despite these obstacles. Closeness and intimacy create enjoyment—a sense of wholeness.

The first step in addressing intimacy is communicating with your partner. You can open the conversation by saying something like, "I miss being close to you," or, "I miss spending time together." Set aside time to be together when you both can be alone and free of interruptions. Turn phones to mute. Turn off the TV and put away anything that may cause distraction. Pay attention to each other and allow time to talk about feelings.

Create an Intimate Atmosphere

- Play music, light candles, and make sure the room is a comfortable temperature.

- Plan time together doing something that you both enjoy, like taking a drive, watching a movie, or reading a book.

- Take a walk together.

Find Ways to Be Intimate

- Talking, caressing, holding hands, and kissing are all ways to be intimate.

- Dim the lights to take the focus off appearance and put the focus on sensation and touch.

- Go slowly.

- Foreplay takes the focus off the act of sex and puts the focus on feeling touch and sensation.

- Try massage, manual stimulation, self-touch, or a vibrator.

- Share a bath or shower.

- Experiment with positions. Use pillows to prop yourself and enhance comfort.

- Allow your partner to take the lead so you can conserve energy.

- Most importantly, keep a sense of humor.

Feeling Fatigued

- Take a nap or rest before spending intimate time with your partner.

- Ask your partner to help with chores.

- Allow your partner to take the active role when being physically intimate.

- Try sharing a bath, shower, or massage.

- Plan to rest after.

Feeling Anxious

- Emotions and physical changes can affect self-esteem. You are no less a man or a woman because of your cancer.

- Talk to a social worker, counselor, or sex therapist.

- If you and your partner are both struggling with your relationship and intimacy, consider seeing a couple's counselor or a marriage counselor. By seeing a counselor together, you may find ways to enhance communication and refresh your relationship.

- Practice pranayama, the breathing exercises described earlier in the book.

- Try guided imagery, focusing on pleasant surroundings. Focus on what it feels like to be loved, physically and emotionally.

- Laugh.

Intercourse During Chemotherapy Treatments

- Chemotherapy can cause a drop in the number of white blood cells, increasing the risk of infection. It can also cause a drop in platelets, increasing the risk of bruising and bleeding. Ask your oncologist or oncology nurse if your blood counts are at a safe level before engaging in intercourse.

- Chemotherapy can increase the risk of birth defects, so it is important to use some form of birth control if there is a risk of pregnancy.

Issues Specific to Women

- Onset of menopause

- Vaginal dryness
  - Low-dose vaginal estrogen replacement may help with vaginal dryness, but its use should be discussed with your oncologist as it may interfere with some medications and may be contraindicated with some types of cancer.
  - Water-based or silicone-based lubricants, vitamin E oil, or coconut oil can be used to make sexual intimacy more comfortable.
  - Vaginal moisturizers should be used at least every other day to help the vaginal tissue regain moisture.
  - A vibrator can restore blood flow and improve elasticity of the vaginal canal.

- Loss of sexual function or sensation
  - Find other ways to be intimate, such as kissing, caressing, massage, or snuggling close.
  - Foreplay and self-touch can get the focus off of the act of having intercourse and put the focus on feeling and sensation.

- Loss of desire

  - Consider speaking with a counselor or sex therapist who can offer support.

  - Communicate with your partner.

  - Plan quality time together doing things you both enjoy to recharge your relationship.

Issues Specific to Men

- Erectile dysfunction (ED)—inability to achieve or maintain an erection

  - Talk with your urologist about erectile dysfunction.

  - Achieving orgasm is possible without achieving erection.

  - Stimulation with hand, mouth, or vibrator can produce an orgasm.

  - Medications can be prescribed to help achieve an erection.

  - A penile vacuum pump is a device that is placed over the penis to increase blood flow and help achieve an erection.

  - Other options include a penile implant or penile injections.

- Incontinence or urine leaking during ejaculation

  - Practice Kegel exercises to strengthen the sphincter muscle responsible for controlling urine. To get started, squeeze the muscles you use to stop urinating midstream. Tighten these muscles and hold for a count of five. Repeat this exercise 10 times throughout the day.

  - Practice Kegel exercises when you are sitting and relaxing, when you are rising from a chair, and when you are about to sneeze or cough.

- Concern about performance or loss of desire
  - Consider joining a men's support group where you can talk to others who are experiencing the same or similar issues.
  - Talk with a counselor or sex therapist.
  - Communicate with your partner.
- Inability to ejaculate (dry ejaculation)
  - Most men can still enjoy climax or orgasm without ejaculation.
- Pain
  - Use a lubricant during intercourse.
  - Try different positions.
  - Let your partner know what makes you comfortable.

Fertility Issues

Cancer treatments can affect fertility. Many women experience early menopause or temporary menopause with chemotherapy. Radiation to the pelvic area can damage organs and cause infertility. Some treatments can lead to decreased hormone levels, making pregnancy difficult.

If pregnancy is something you are considering in your future, talk with your treatment team prior to starting treatment. Ask for a referral to a reproductive specialist who can walk you through options for preserving fertility.

Men may want to consider sperm banking, also known as sperm cryopreservation. Sperm banks can provide kits for collecting a semen sample. The lab will then do an analysis to count the number of active sperm. If the sperm count is high enough, the sperm are frozen for future use. Sperm can be kept frozen for 20 years or more.

Women have a few options when considering fertility preservation. Eggs can be collected and frozen in a procedure called oocyte cryopreservation. Surgery or radiation therapy may be done in such a way as to avoid harming reproductive organs. Hormone treatments can also be considered to suppress the activity of the ovaries until treatment is complete.

LIVESTRONG provides information, resources, and brochures to support cancer patients and survivors with fertility issues. Since many insurance companies do not cover fertility preservation, LIVESTRONG can provide information and support to obtain financial assistance. Visit www.livestrong.org or call 855-844-7777 to speak with a navigator.

Oncolink (www.oncolink.org) provides a guide to sexuality for both men and women. You can also find additional sources of information and support on their website. US Too is an organization that provides education and support for men, and their loved ones, who are affected by prostate cancer. You can find information on treatment side effects, including erectile dysfunction, by visiting www.ustoo.org or calling 800-808-7866.

Will2Love (www.will2love.com) is a website created by a clinical psychologist who is an expert on sexual problems and infertility related to cancer treatment. The website provides information, news, forums, webinars, and resources on topics related to sexuality and parenthood. Will2Love also offers online self-help programs and telehealth coaching and counseling. Call 832-644-0406 for more information.

Cancer throws many obstacles that make it difficult to focus on intimacy and sexuality. But you are no less a man or a woman because of your cancer. Many strategies can help you navigate around these obstacles and through your cancer treatments. You deserve to be loved and feel loved.

Chapter 10

If Cancer Recurs

Physicians take great care in mapping out a treatment plan that is patient-specific and intended to produce the best results. But cancer is not an exact science and, even with the best intentions, there is no way of predicting how things will turn out. Cancer may recur at the site of origin, or it may metastasize, spreading to other areas of the body. Sometimes tumors that were stable may start to grow.

Hearing that your cancer has progressed or did not respond to treatment is difficult. You may feel all those same feelings you had when you were first diagnosed—shock, disbelief, fear, anger, and disappointment. The decision-making process starts all over again, but you may find that your goals and wishes have changed.

A diagnosis of cancer certainly makes us think about our mortality, regardless of the stage. When cancer progresses, thoughts of mortality are front and center. But remember that disease progression does not mean death is around the corner. Cancer is a chronic disease, like diabetes or asthma. Many people live years with advanced cancer. Many people live a fulfilling life in spite of their disease. The difference is the focus changes from cure to control.

Oncologists have an expanding arsenal of treatment options at their ready. This is an exciting time as our understanding of cancer and genetics is growing. Surgery, chemotherapy, immunotherapy, targeted therapy, radiation, and clinical trials may be part of the options offered to you. But, ultimately, the decision rests with you. Obtain second and third opinions, if you desire. Discuss all of your options with your cancer care team, but do not allow anyone to make decisions for you. This is your cancer and your life, and you decide how you want to live it. It can be empowering to be able to choose.

Coping with Disease Recurrence

- **Acceptance**: You may question what you could have done to avoid recurrence. You may ask, "Why me and why now?" Avoid blaming yourself. Instead, ask "What can I do from here to live the life I choose?"

- **Set goals**: Ask yourself, "What are my goals, hopes, and values?" For some, this may include pursuing all avenues of treatment available. For others, this may mean comfort and quality over quantity of life.

- **Learn from the past**: What worked for you? How did you cope?

- **Seek support**: Support groups, counselors, religious leaders, and chaplains are all sources of support. Sharing your feelings with others is helpful.

- **Nurture your spirit**: What gives your life meaning? What brings you joy?

- **Communicate with your oncologist**: Discuss your wishes with your oncologist. It may help to ask the following questions before making a treatment decision:
  - What treatment options are available to me?
  - What are the possible side effects of these options?
  - What can I expect from treatment?
  - Is the goal to get rid of the cancer, stabilize my disease, or control symptoms?
  - What is my expected prognosis with and without treatment?

- **Talk with family and loved ones**: Let them know your wishes and how they can support you. Part of the decision-making process may involve difficult conversations. Family and loved ones may have different opinions regarding your care. They may have difficulty dealing with their own emotions. Talking about your wishes may take away some of their uncertainties and fears and strengthen relationships. This is an opportunity to plan for the future, decide how you want to live, and put your life in order.

Advance Directives

One of the best ways to ensure that your wishes are respected, is to address advance directives. Advance directives include a living will and a health care proxy. A living will is a document that allows you to determine the extent of medical care you wish to receive should you be unable to make your own medical decisions. A health care proxy is a directive that allows you to select a person, or persons, you entrust with making medical or end-of-life decisions on your behalf. The best time to address advance directives is when you are feeling well.

It may not be an easy topic to introduce to loved ones, but it can take a huge burden off family and friends, and it allows you the power to make your wishes known. The National Hospice and Palliative Care Organization offers a wealth of information about advance directives at www.caringinfo.org. The site gives a clear explanation of advance directives and has a link to download forms that are specific to the state in which you reside. You may also want to make a list of personal information that others may need to know—bank information, passwords, and location of important documents. Many people express a peace of mind in putting this information in order.

Palliative Care

Palliative care is a program designed for people living with chronic disease. The focus is on managing symptoms of the disease and treatment side effects to enhance quality of daily life. Palliative care provides emotional support to you and your loved ones and can help you set goals for the future. You can request a referral to palliative care at any time and at any stage of cancer. Palliative care serves as an adjunct to your physician's care. It allows your oncologist to focus on your treatment and the palliative care team to focus on your symptoms.

Choosing No More Treatment

What if you do not want to continue cancer treatment? It does not mean that you are giving up or losing hope. Perhaps your goals and hopes have changed, and you now value quality over quantity of life. Choosing to have no treatment is your option to choose. Palliative care is available to help support you emotionally and physically.

If your cancer is no longer responding to treatment, and your oncologist feels you have a limited life expectancy of 6 months or less, you may begin to think about how and where you would like to spend your last days. Hospice is an option. Hospice provides care to those who have opted against further treatment. The focus is on enhancing one's quality of life with dignity and compassion. Family and loved ones gain much support from hospice. Care is usually provided in the comfort of one's home, although some programs have in-patient facilities. Because quality of life is improved, people often live longer with hospice. A hospice team may include doctors, nurses, social workers, home health aides, chaplains, and respite care. Hospice can also provide medications to manage symptoms and equipment to make your home safe and give you more independence. Hospice services are covered by Medicare, Medicaid, and private insurance. Communicate your wishes with your oncologist. If you choose hospice, your oncologist will need to make a referral on your behalf.

Making Choices

Talk with your cancer care team about your treatment options. Consider a second or third opinion. Obtain as much information as you need to make a decision regarding your care. Talk with your family and loved ones about your wishes. Think about your values and reframe your goals. Make a treatment decision that is in line with those values and goals.

No matter what decision you make, do not forget to take care of your mental and spiritual health. Counselors, support groups, chaplains, and religious leaders can help you deal with fear, anger, and sadness. They can give you direction to help make decisions. You may want to review previous chapters on caring for your spirit and dealing with stress and depression. Your loved ones may also benefit from additional support at this time.

Cancer forces you to face mortality. Facing death and accepting its possibility is not surrendering, or quitting, or giving up hope. Death is part of the natural course of all living creatures. When death is viewed as an inevitable part of life, it can diminish fear and make conversations easier. It offers a chance to plan how life's journey is traveled. Take time to strengthen relationships and enjoy simple pleasures. No matter where you are in your cancer journey, take advantage of the chance to live the way you choose.

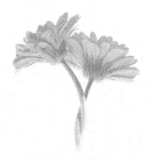

Part V

Life Beyond Cancer

Chapter 11

Moving Forward

The road from diagnosis through treatment completion is a long and emotional one. Once the day arrives, there is a sense of accomplishment and relief. This is a time for joyous celebration!

Many people reach this milestone and are ready to move on. But many more people are surprised to find this day, so eagerly anticipated, is fraught with mixed emotions. Recovery from cancer treatment does not happen with a snap of the fingers. It is a gradual process. Physical and emotional changes may linger for months. A lot of energy has been directed at getting through treatment. Now that treatment is complete, it is time to process the experience and reassess goals and values. Cancer changes you in ways you may have never imagined. Adjusting to your new normal and transitioning back into the world takes time.

You may feel as if you are on an emotional roller coaster. Happiness, gratitude, and relief may be mixed with anxiety, fear, and sadness. Frequent medical appointments become less frequent and you are expected to go back to your normal routine. But cancer is a chronic disease and it is not so easy to pick up where you left off. You may grieve the loss of support from your doctors, nurses, friends and family. Side effects, such as fatigue, pain, sexual dysfunction, and cognitive issues may linger. You may worry about cancer recurrence. All of these feelings are a normal part of transitioning from patient to survivor.

Seven Essential Strategies to Help You Transition

1. **Communicate** with family and friends.

2. **Be patient** with yourself and with others.

3. **Connect** with other cancer survivors.

4. **Address fears and emotions that may arise.**

5. **Collaborate** with your oncologist to develop a survivorship care plan.

6. **Nurture** your spirit, mind, and body.

7. **Give yourself permission** to move forward.

Communicate with Friends and Family

Well-meaning friends and family may expect you to resume your life where you left off. Roles and household responsibilities may have changed while you were undergoing treatment and redefining roles can be difficult when treatment ends. Family and friends may not understand that recovery takes time and you may need their support as you continue to recover. Let them know how you feel and what they can—and cannot—expect of you.

Be Patient with Yourself and Others

Relationships can change throughout cancer treatment. You may find some relationships become stronger, while others may have dwindled off. Surround yourself with positive, supportive people who can encourage you as you continue to heal and recover.

Connect with Other Cancer Survivors

Talking with others can be uplifting when they can relate to your experiences and validate your feelings. Support groups can provide a safe environment where survivors can talk face-to-face and cultivate friendships. Not everyone feels comfortable talking in a group. Support group meetings can also conflict with work and appointments. In this case, online cancer survivor groups can be beneficial. The Cancer Support Community organization provides message boards where you can post questions, comments, and words of support. Visit the site at www.cancersupportcommunity. org and click on the *Find Support* tab.

Address Fears and Emotions

Once treatment is finished, visits to the doctor decrease. The comfort of knowing someone is looking out for you is suddenly gone. For many, the relief of having completed treatment is replaced by fear of recurrence. An unusual ache, pain, or cough; news of a friend, relative, or celebrity's cancer experience; medical appointments and follow-up tests can be anxiety triggers. For me, every back ache, every new mole, and every visit to my dermatology surgeon triggers anxiety over possible recurrence. The fear and anxiety may never completely go away, but the worry will lighten as time progresses. Coping strategies can help prepare you for anxiety triggers. The following tips may help you address your fears:

- **Acknowledge** your fear without judgment.
- **Talk** with your cancer care team about your fears and ask what signs and symptoms warrant a call.
- **Call** your doctor to report any symptoms that are unusual or worrisome. Do not let fear prevent you from addressing a concern. A phone call may be all it takes to put your mind at ease.
- **Connect** with other cancer survivors.
- **Support** from family, friends, counselors, and chaplains can be a source of comfort.
- **Mindfulness** techniques—meditation, guided imagery, yoga, deep breathing—are just as helpful now as they were when you were going through treatment.
- **Attach** a pleasant experience to your follow up appointments. It could be as simple as planning a stop at a favorite café or coffee shop on the way home or taking the scenic route and stopping for a walk.

Many people wonder how they held it together through treatment, but feel like their world is falling apart once treatment is complete. Overwhelming sadness, anger, and guilt can leave a hollow feeling inside. Many cancer patients report feeling down, or having the blues, once treatment is complete. When the blues lead to depression, it creates an invisible wall between being the cancer patient and transitioning back into the world.

If you experience two or more of the following symptoms, and they have lasted more than two weeks, you may be suffering from post-treatment depression:

- Worry or anxiety that interferes with daily activities
- Feelings of sadness or hopelessness that interfere with relationships and prevent you from engaging in social activities
- Decreased energy and motivation
- Sleeping more than usual or difficulty falling asleep
- Difficulty focusing or making decisions
- Feelings of hopelessness

The same methods used to heal depression during treatment can be used in the recovery phase. A chaplain, social worker, or mental health counselor will offer an objective, nonjudgmental ear. Support groups can help validate your feelings and facilitate moving forward.

Talk with your health care provider about your depression. Some medications prescribed post-treatment, such as hormone modifiers, can cause or exacerbate depression. Your physician can help evaluate whether your depression is related to your medication. Sometimes, a change in medication can lift the depression. Your physician will also be able to refer you to a counselor who can help you work through your feelings.

As discussed earlier in this book, depression is not a sign of weakness. It can't be turned off and on at will. Depression is a medical condition related to a chemical imbalance in the brain. Medication, when coupled with counseling, can help lift depression and create emotional balance so you can be empowered to move forward.

Collaborate on a Survivorship Care Plan

Throughout this book, we have talked about being empowered, proactive, and prepared. As you transition into survivorship, it is crucial that you continue being empowered, proactive, and prepared. Your continued health and wellbeing are of the utmost concern, so having a plan for moving forward is essential. One way to do that is to develop a survivorship care plan with your cancer care team. A care plan creates a history of your treatments and details a plan for follow up. It helps answer the question, What do I do next?

The first thing to include in the care plan is a copy of your history and physical. Your oncologist can provide this for you. It will detail your diagnosis, stage, tests that were done, and treatment that you received. It will summarize the details of your cancer history and help you and your oncologist develop your survivorship care plan.

Since the survivorship care plan is a road map to guide you in caring for yourself post-treatment, it should include answers to the following questions:

- What long-term side effects can I expect? How long will they last?
- Who should I follow up with and how often?
- What tests will be done as part of my follow up? Who will order these tests? How often will I have them done?
- What lab work should I be having as part of my follow up? Who will order my labs and how often will they be done?

- What symptoms should I be aware of and what symptoms should I report?
- Who should I call if I have a symptom that concerns me?
- What screening or preventive tests should I have? Who will order these?
- What can I do to optimize my health?

Some cancer treatment centers offer a survivorship program to help you make a healthy transition from treatment. The program consists of an appointment with a nurse practitioner, your physician, and a social worker or counselor. Some centers also include a visit with a dietitian and a referral to a cancer rehabilitation program. Your medical history will be reviewed, you will be referred for screening tests, and you will receive information on healthy living habits. The team will develop a survivorship care plan to guide you in your transition.

Journey Forward is an organization whose goal is to improve the care of cancer survivors. They have developed several tools to help patients and health care professionals address the challenges of cancer survivors. Their website contains a library of resources to help patients transition into survivorship. They also offer care plan builders that are downloadable to computer or smart phone. You can visit their site at www.journeyforward.org.

Nurture Your Spirit, Mind, and Body

By nurturing the spirit, mind, and body, you can regain control and choose how you want to live your life going forward. Earlier in the book, we talked about the effects spirituality can have in creating physical wellbeing and inner peace while undergoing cancer treatment. We also talked about the powerful healing effects of nutrition and physical activity. Spirituality, nutrition, and physical activity should continue to be priorities.

Now that treatment is finished, you may want to revisit earlier questions regarding spirituality:

- What gives my life meaning?
- What gives me a sense of purpose?
- What helps me connect with others?
- What connects me to nature?
- How do I connect with myself?
- What do I value?
- What brings me peace? Joy? Love?

Have your answers changed? What would help you nurture your spirit and your mind?

Now think about what would help you nourish your body. Whole food nutrition provides your body with more energy, a more robust immune system, and quicker healing and recovery. If you continue to be challenged by taste changes or swallowing difficulties, you may want to talk with a dietitian who can address those issues and help you develop a plan for healthy eating now that treatment is finished. Review the chapter on whole food nutrition. Try new foods and new recipes and feed your body the fuel it needs to stay healthy.

What you do with your body is just as important as what you put in your body. Physical activity has been associated with lower risk of recurrence and increased survival after cancer treatment. Exercise also improves mood, decreases risk of depression, and lowers the risk of other conditions like diabetes and heart disease. If you were not physically active prior to treatment, start slowly, but start something. Exercise should be enjoyable and should not put stress or strain on your joints. Try swimming, resistance bands, water aerobics, gentle yoga, walking, or biking. If you need motivation, enroll in a class or grab an exercise buddy who can offer encouragement and support. Some hospitals and cancer centers offer cancer rehabilitation classes. Your oncologist will be able to make a referral.

If you were active prior to treatment, understand that you may need to readjust your expectations. Set small, achievable goals and increase those goals slowly. Exercise when you feel your energy is at its best.

Give Yourself Permission

Whether you are deemed cancer-free or have stable disease, you have come far. You have endured tests, doctor visits, treatment, symptoms, and side effects, all the while managing everything that goes along with managing life. You are all of these—fighter, trooper, soldier, hero, victor, champion, thriver, and survivor.

Life is such a gift. Each and every day should be lived fully. Give yourself permission to find joy in each day. Give yourself permission to move forward. Set off on a new adventure. Try something you have never tried before. Continue to care for your spirit, mind, and body.

- Practice mindfulness
- Nourish your spirit
- Connect with other cancer survivors

- Volunteer
- Join a club
- Take a class
- Explore
- Exercise
- Eat a whole foods diet
- Meditate
- Write, draw, paint, create
- Immerse yourself in nature
- Sing and dance
- Listen to music
- Make music
- Learn something new
- Travel
- Do something you have dreamed of doing

You are a beautiful being. You are strong and you have come so far. Love yourself and care for yourself. Go forward and know you are a bright shining star that illuminates the sky. Take small steps every day as you navigate forward and create a new chapter. Always stay *Empowered, Proactive,* and *Prepared.*

Appendix A

Glossary

absolute neutrophil count (ANC): Doctors use ANC to determine risk of infection. ANC is found by multiplying the number of white blood cells (WBC) by the percent of neutrophils.

adjuvant treatment: Treatment given in addition to the primary, initial treatment. It usually refers to treatment given after surgery to reduce the risk of recurrence.

allogeneic transplant: A procedure in which a person receives stem cells or bone marrow from a genetically similar donor. This could be a family member or an unrelated donor.

alopecia: The loss of hair in an area that previously had hair growth.

alternative treatment: Medical products and therapies used in place of standard or conventional treatment. Examples include herbs, homeopathy, mega doses of vitamins, and acupuncture.

anemia: The condition of having a lower than normal number of red blood cells.

antiemetic: A medication or therapy used to prevent or treat nausea and vomiting.

arthralgia: Joint pain.

autologous transplant: A procedure in which a person's own stem cells or bone marrow is collected, stored, and then reinfused after the person is treated with high-dose chemotherapy or radiation.

cellulitis: A bacterial skin infection that appears as a red, tender, swollen area.

clinical trial: A research study in which a medication, treatment, or device is tested to evaluate side effects and benefits to humans.

complementary therapy: The use of healing products or therapies that address the mind-body connection. Examples include yoga, aromatherapy, reiki, therapeutic touch.

conventional treatment: This is also known as allopathic treatment, Western medicine, or standard treatment. It is focused on the diagnosis and treatment of illness and disease and is administered by a healthcare professional.

co-pay: A fixed amount of money you pay for a health care service. This amount can vary depending on the service or prescription being filled.

cure: A person no longer requires cancer treatment and their risk of recurrence mirrors that of the general population.

deductible: The amount you will be expected to pay out-of-pocket before your insurance begins to pay.

dysphagia: Difficulty swallowing or painful swallowing.

edema: An abnormal build-up of fluid under the skin that occurs most commonly in the hands, arms, feet, and legs.

endocrine therapy: To slow or stop the growth of certain hormone-sensitive cancers by using a medication or surgery to block a particular hormone that feeds the cancer, also known as *hormone therapy.*

esophagitis: An inflammation of the esophagus or throat.

HMO: The acronym stands for Health Maintenance Organization. Care under an HMO plan is covered only if you see an in-network physician. There are no out-of-network benefits. Most HMO plans require that you choose a primary care physician (PCP) and obtain a written referral before seeing a specialist.

hypertension: Also known as high blood pressure. It occurs when the force of blood pumping through your veins is too high.

hyperglycemia: An excessive amount of glucose circulating in the blood.

hypoglycemia: An abnormally low level of glucose in the blood.

insurance premium: The amount a person pays each month for their insurance.

integrative medicine: A holistic type of medicine that focuses on mental, physical, emotional, and spiritual aspects of a person. It combines complementary or alternative treatment with conventional treatment.

lymph fluid: Clear fluid that flows through the lymphatic system. It carries infection-fighting cells.

lymphedema: An abnormal buildup of lymph fluid in fatty tissue beneath the skin.

metastasis: The spread of cancer cells from their place of origin to another place in the body.

mucositis: Inflammation of the mucus membranes of the digestive tract. It may involve the mouth, throat, stomach, and intestines.

myalgia: Muscle aches.

nadir. The point at which the blood counts are at their lowest after cancer treatment. White blood cells usually reach their nadir 7-10 days after chemotherapy administration.

neoadjuvant treatment: The first course of treatment given to shrink a tumor before surgery.

neutrophil: A type of white blood cell that fights infection.

neutropenia: A lower than normal amount of infection-fighting neutrophils, increasing the risk of infection. It is determined by an ANC less than 1500.

palliation/palliative care: Treatment focused on controlling symptoms and providing comfort and quality of life.

peripheral neuropathy: Some chemotherapy drugs can damage the nerves in the hands and feet. People with peripheral neuropathy may experience numbness, tingling, pain, or cold sensitivity in the fingers, hands, toes, and/or feet.

PPO: This acronym stands for Preferred Physician Organization and refers to an insurance plan that allows the insured to choose physicians from a list of network providers.

pranayama: Exercises and techniques that bring awareness to the breath thereby increasing energy and facilitating relaxation.

religion: A set of beliefs and practices within an organized group.

remission: In partial remission, there is a decrease in signs and symptoms of cancer. In complete remission, all tests, scans, and physical exams show no signs of cancer.

spirituality: A sense of being connected to self, nature, and others. It is also a belief that there exists a power greater than oneself.

stable disease: No signs of tumor growth or shrinkage and no signs of new tumors.

stomatitis: Inflammation and soreness of the mouth.

thrombocytopenia: A platelet count that falls below normal levels. It may cause prolonged bleeding and bruising.

thrush: A fungal infection in the mouth characterized by white patches or white coating on the gums and tongue.

Appendix B

Nutrition Tips and Suggestions

Essential Kitchen Tools

- **Blender**—A blender is ideal for making soups, smoothies, shakes, and sauces. It is also great for pureeing food if chewing and swallowing are difficult.

- **Crockpot**—Ingredients for soup, stew, chili, casseroles, meat, or poultry dishes can be thrown in a crockpot and left to cook for several hours. A crock pot helps make fuss-free meals and provides several servings for the week.

- **Toaster oven**—Although microwaves are convenient, they tend to enhance the odor of whatever is being heated. If you find you are sensitive to strong odors, you may want to try heating food in a toaster oven.

- **Mason jars**—Overnight oatmeal, individual salads, and yogurt parfaits can be easily portioned into a mason jar. The jars provide a single-serving and are portable enough to take with you for a quick meal or snack.

- **Ice pop molds**—Pureed fruit, prepared smoothies, coconut water, and yogurt can all be frozen into ice pop molds for a healthy snack. Ice pops can be a great way to increase hydration and they also help soothe a tender mouth and throat.

- **Ice cube trays**—Use an ice cube tray to freeze juice or electrolyte drinks. You can also freeze chopped fruit, which can be used to make smoothies.

Make Meal Preparation Easier

- Vegetables
  - Wash, cut, and portion them into individual containers or baggies to store in the freezer.
  - Add to broth with noodles and protein for a quick soup.
  - Puree in a blender with broth and add yogurt, cream, milk or non-dairy milk for a creamed soup.
  - Top a baked potato or sweet potato with steamed vegetables.
  - Add to an omelet.

- Fruit
  - Wash, cut, and portion into containers to make a quick fruit salad.
  - Wash, cut, and portion into individual containers or baggies and store in the freezer. Add frozen fruit to shakes or smoothies.
  - Add fruit to yogurt or oatmeal.

- Whole grains
  - Make a batch of rice, barley, quinoa, or other whole grain and keep in the refrigerator.
  - Add grains to soup, chili, or stew.
  - Top grains with beans or lean protein. Add gravy, olive oil and vinegar, or tomato sauce. Top with cheese.
- Double up recipes and store in individual portions.
- Use mason jars to layer pasta, protein, cooked vegetables, and dressing for a quick lunch or dinner.
- Store pancakes and muffins in the freezer and reheat in the toaster oven.

Tricks for Adding Calories

- Add mashed potato flakes to creamy soups or stews.
- Canned coconut milk adds healthy fat and calories to smoothies and creamy soups.
- Powdered milk can be added to scrambled eggs, pancake batter, smoothies, creamed soups, and gravies for a boost of protein and calories.
- Avocadoes are high in calories and are nutrient-dense. Because they have a neutral taste, they can easily be blended into a smoothie or a creamed soup. They can be added to sandwiches, used as a topping on baked potatoes, or pureed with yogurt and herbs for a dip. You can also use avocadoes as a base for making pudding.
- Soak raw cashews in water overnight. Puree the cashews in soup or smoothies to add richness, nutrients, and calories.

Electrolyte Drink

Many commercial electrolyte replacement sports drinks contain artificial colors and ingredients. You can make your own electrolyte drink and store it in the refrigerator. You can also pour the drink into an ice cube tray and suck on the cubes if you are nauseas or have diarrhea.

Electrolyte Drink 1
- 1 quart water
- ½ teaspoon baking soda
- ½ teaspoon salt
- 1 tablespoon sweetener of choice

Mix well and store in a container in the refrigerator.

Electrolyte Drink 2
- 3 ½ cups water
- ½ cup grape or apple juice
- 2 ½ tablespoons sweetener of choice
- ¼ teaspoon salt

Mix well and store in a container in the refrigerator.

Basic Smoothie Recipe
(Single serving)

Your base consists of 1 cup greens, 1 ½ cup fruit, and 1 cup liquid. Below are some ideas for ingredients. Feel free to mix it up and be creative. Skip the greens, if you want. Add extra fruit or liquid. Adding ice cubes gives it a shake-like consistency. Experiment with these ingredients and portions.

Green Options
- Spinach
- Kale
- Avocado
- Carrots, canned pumpkin, cooked butternut squash (not technically greens, but they sweeten up a smoothie)

Fruit Options
You can use any combination of fresh, canned, or frozen fruit.

If you are neutropenic, make sure you only use fruit that can be peeled.
- Banana
- Berries
- Papaya
- Mango
- Pineapple
- Cherries
- Apple

Liquid Options
- Almond, soy, cashew milk
- Full fat coconut milk
- Dairy milk
- Coconut water
- Water
- Fruit juice

Options for Add-ins
- Ground flax seeds or flax seed oil
- Chia seeds

- Greek yogurt
- Peanut, almond, cashew, or sunflower butter
- Peanut butter powder
- Protein powder
- Cinnamon, vanilla, turmeric, cocoa powder

Overnight Oatmeal Recipe
(Single serving)

Basic Overnight Oatmeal

- 1 cup nut milk, coconut milk, or dairy milk
- ½ cup rolled oats
- 1 tablespoon maple syrup

Options for Add-ins

- 1 tablespoon chia seeds or ground flax seeds
- 2 tablespoons nut butter (peanut, almond, cashew, sunflower)
- 2 tablespoons peanut butter powder
- 1 scoop protein powder
- ½-1/3 cup Greek yogurt
- ½ mashed banana
- ½ cup chopped or dried fruit
- 1 tablespoon chopped nuts

Add all ingredients to a mason jar. Stir or shake. Cover and refrigerate overnight. Eat straight from the jar.

Avocado Pudding Recipe

- 1 large avocado, chopped
- 3 tablespoons unsweetened cocoa powder

- 3 tablespoons brown sugar or maple syrup
- 6 tablespoons coconut, almond, or soy milk

Puree in a blender, then chill until ready to eat.

Chia Pudding Recipe

Chia seeds are rich in omega-3 fatty acids, as well as antioxidants. They add a crunch when sprinkled on salad, yogurt, or cereal. But the real magic is when they are added to a liquid. Chia seeds absorb liquid and transform into a gel-like pudding. The recipe couldn't be easier to make and can be stored in the refrigerator for a healthy snack.

- 1 cup dairy or non-dairy milk
- 3 tablespoons chia seeds
- 1-2 teaspoons maple syrup, agave nectar, or honey
- Cinnamon, vanilla extract, cocoa powder, if desired

Add all ingredients to a mason jar. Shake well. Store in the refrigerator for at least 8 hours. Stir to break up any clumps before eating.

Soothing Miso Soup

- 1 cup water or broth
- 1 tablespoon miso paste

Stir until miso is dissolved. For a heartier soup add any combination of the following:

- Cooked pasta
- Frozen mixed vegetables
- Mushrooms

- Spinach
- Cubed cooked chicken, diced cooked shrimp, edamame, or cubed tofu

Ginger Tea

- 2 cups water
- 1-inch piece of ginger root cut into thin slices
- 2 herbal or green tea bags (optional)
- 1 tablespoon sweetener of choice

Bring water to a boil. Add ginger root and tea bags, if desired. Turn off heat, cover, and let steep for 10 minutes. Add sweetener. Pour into a mug and sip.

Appendix C

Resources

Cancer Care Plans

- www.journeyforward.org Journey Forward provides tools for creating your own cancer care plan. The site also provides information on patient tools that can be downloaded to your smart phone.

Clinical Trials

- www.clinicaltrials.gov (1-800-4-CANCER) A service of the U.S. National Institute of Health allows patients and physicians to search for clinical trials around the world.

Complementary and Alternative Health Care Information

- www.nccih.nih.gov The National Center for Complementary and Integrative Health is a service of the National Institute of Health. The site provides information about complementary health products and practices, including a database listing of herbs and supplements.

Create a Blog or Journal Online

- **www.caringbridge.org.** Create a free personal website to keep friends and loved ones updated on your condition.

- **www.cancersupportcommunity.org** Click on the *Find Support* link. Then click on *The Living Room*. Scroll down to *My LifeLine* to create a personal blog or webpage.

Employment Questions

- **www.cancerandcareers.org** Cancer and Careers provides expert advice to educate cancer patients about work and employment. Their services include information on working through treatment, career coaching, and free resume reviews.

- **www.dol.gov** Click on *Topics* in the Department of Labor website and find information on employment rights and resources. You can learn more about COBRA (Continuation of Health Coverage), disability resources, and FMLA (Family and Medical Leave).

- **www.patientadvocate.org (1-800-532-5274)** Patient Advocate provides a wealth of resources to help cancer patients find financial assistance, information on employment and job retention, and help with medical debt.

Fertility

- **www.fertilehope.org (1-800-844-777)** Live Strong provides education for cancer patients whose fertility may be compromised by cancer treatment. They also provide financial assistance for fertility medications and procedures related to fertility and reproduction.

- www.will2love.com **(832-644-0406)** News, resources, and telehealth coaching are just some of the services provided to cancer survivors interested in becoming parents.

Financial Resources

- **www.cancer.org (1-800-227-2345)** American Cancer Society offers information to help you deal with financial and insurance issues. Click on *Treatment & Support*, then *Finding & Paying for Treatment.*

- **www.copays.org** The Patient Advocate Foundation's Co-Pay Relief Program provides financial assistance to help pay with the co-payments and premiums on cancer treatment medications.

- **www.cancercare.org (1-800-813-4673)** CancerCare can provide limited financial assistance to help pay for transportation, lymphedema supplies, medical equipment, and certain medications. The organization also provides social workers who can assist in finding additional resources.

- **www.cancerfac.org** Enter your zip code, cancer type, and the type of assistance you are looking for, and this website will provide a customized list of resources. You can search for transportation, medication assistance, housing, insurance, and financial assistance.

- **www.211.org (Call 211)** This is a free, confidential service that finds local resources to help with housing, food, health care, as well as disaster and crisis intervention.

- **www.panfoundation.org (1-866-316-7263)** The Patient Advocate Network (PAN) Foundation works with underinsured patients living with chronic and rare diseases to help them get obtain financial assistance so they can have access to the care they need.

- **www.patientadvocate.org (1-800-532-5274)** Patient Advocate provides a wealth of resources to help cancer patients find financial assistance, information on employment and job retention, and help with medical debt.

General Cancer Information

- **www.cancer.org (1-800-227-2345)** American Cancer Society provides information on specific cancers, treatment, and side effect management. The site also provides information on the latest research.

- **www.cancer.gov (1-800-4-CANCER)** The National Cancer Institute also provides information on specific cancers, treatment, and research. You can also order free publications from their extensive library.

- **www.nccn.org** The National Comprehensive Cancer Network is an alliance of cancer centers whose goal is to provide quality care to cancer patients through research and education. Click on *NCCN Guidelines* to access a list of treatment guidelines to help patients understand their treatment options.

- **www.cancer.net** Developed by the American Society of Clinical Oncology (ASCO), this site provides resources for cancer patients to learn more about their type of cancer. The site also provides information on coping with cancer and on survivorship.

- **www.chemocare.com** Scott Hamilton, Olympic Figure Skating Champion, is the brain-child behind Chemocare. The site provides easy to understand information on chemotherapy and side effect management.

Insurance Information
- **www.healthcare.gov (1-800-318-2596)** This is the official website of the Affordable Care Act. Individuals can search for health care coverage options.

Living Wills and Advance Directives
- **www.caringinfo.org** A program of the National Hospice and Palliative Care Organization provides information on caregiving, advanced care planning, palliative care, and hospice.

- **www.cancer.net** Click on the *Navigating Cancer* link, then click on *Advanced Cancer* for information on end-of-life planning.

Magazines
- **www.curetoday.com** Visit the CURE website for the latest news and articles to help support you through your cancer journey. You can also order a free subscription to CURE magazine, a source of support for cancer patients, survivors, and caregivers.

- **www.copingmag.com** Order a free subscription to *Coping with Cancer* magazine.

- **www.conquer-magazine.com** Read articles online or order a free subscription to the official patient magazine of the Academy of Oncology Nurse & Patient Navigators (AONN).

Topics include survivorship, healthy living, financial support, and patient stories.

- **www.awomanshealth.com** Access articles covering women's health, wellness, nutrition, and cancer.

Medication and Drug Discounts

- **www.pparx.org** The Partnership for Prescription Assistance offers a single point of access to help low-income and uninsured patients get free or low-cost medications.

- **www.needymeds.com** Find prescription assistance, free or low-cost medical and dental clinics, medication coupons, scholarships, and camps.

- **www.rxassist.org** RxAssist provides information on obtaining free and low cost medication.

Mindfulness and Meditation

- **www.buddhify.com** Buddhify is accessible through your mobile device. It is home to theme-based guided meditations to help manage stress and facilitate sleep.

- **www.headspace.com** Headspace provides hundreds of themed meditations, including meditations for busy schedules and meditations guides.

- **www.insighttimer.com** Guided meditations, podcasts, and meditation communities are available in this free application for your mobile device.

- **www.thisiskara.com** Kara contains guided meditations designed to assist those affected by cancer.

Nutrition

- **www.myfitnesspal.com** My Fitness Pal helps you reach a healthy weight tracking your food choices and daily exercise.

- **http://www.aicr.org/assets/docs/pdf/education/heal-well-guide.pdf** A joint venture of the American Institute for Cancer Research (AICR), LiveStrong Foundation, and Savor Your Health, provides information about diet, nutrition and exercise during and after cancer treatment. It also provides information to help manage eating-related issues.

- **www.pcrm.org** On Physicians Committee for Responsible Medicine's website, click on the *Health and Nutrition* link to find recipes, breaking medical news, information on vegan and vegetarian diets, diabetes resources, and nutrition information for specific diseases.

Sexuality

- **www.ustoo.org (1-800-808-7866)** Us TOO offers peer-to-peer support and educational materials to men and their loved ones affected by prostate cancer. Click on *Prostate Cancer,* then *Side Effects* for information on managing erectile dysfunction and impotence.

- **www.will2love.com (832-644-0406)** Free educational forums, webinars, resources, and coaching are offered to guide cancer patients towards sexual wellness and parenthood.

- **www.oncolink.org** Click on the *Patients* tab. Then click on *Sexuality and Fertility* under the *Support* heading.

Social Security Programs

- **Medicare**

  ○ **www.medicare.gov (1-800-633-4227)** This is the official government site for Medicare.

  ○ **www.mymedicarematters.org** National Council on Aging's Medicare Matters website helps take the complexity out of understanding your Medicare options.

  ○ **www.mymedicare.gov** Access personalized information about your Medicare benefits. There is an option to do a live chat or take a virtual tour.

- **Medicaid**

  ○ **www.healthcare.gov (1-800-318-2596)** Click on the link *Get Coverage* to obtain information and to apply for Medicaid.

- **SSDI & SSI**

  ○ **www.ssa.gov (1-800-772-1213)** Find out about Social Security benefits on this government website.

Support Communities

- **www.cancersupportcommunity.org (1-888-793-9355)** Find support through their toll-free help line, live web chat, or online communities. You can also search for local support groups by entering your zip code.

- **www.cancercare.org (1-800-813-4673)** CancerCare offers counseling, support, education, and financial assistance. Cancer patients and their caregivers can call the toll-free number to speak with an oncology social worker.

- **www.inspire.com** This support community offers education, support, and opportunities to share with others who are dealing with a chronic illness.

- **www.friend4life.org** This organization will match both cancer patients and caregivers with someone who has experienced a cancer or treatment similar to yours for one-on-one support.

Wigs and Alopecia Resources

- **www.lookgoodfeelbetter.com (1-800-395-LOOK)** Look Good Feel Better programs teach beauty techniques to women undergoing cancer treatment. Workshops are held throughout the year at locations across the United States. Visit the website or call to find a workshop near you.

- **www.tlcdirect.org (1-800-850-9445)** Browse the American Cancer Society's catalogue of low-cost wigs, head coverings, mastectomy products, and cancer support jewelry.

- **www.rapunzelproject.org** The Rapunzel Project is dedicated to helping chemotherapy patients keep their hair by providing up-to-date information on cold cap therapy.

- **www.hairtostay.org** This organization is dedicated to providing financial support to patients who are not able to afford cold cap therapy.

Acknowledgments

My heartfelt thanks to the following people who inspired me, believed in me, and assisted me in the writing of *The By-Your-Side Cancer Guide:*

Howard Gomer, my husband, who planted the seed to write this book. His encouragement and belief in me were the juice I needed to write every day.

Lawrence Solomon, my father, who also planted the seed to write this book. His unwavering support pushed me to see this book to fruition.

Deborrah Hoag, my editor. Her advice, critiques, and suggestions have made me a better writer. I knew we would make a great team from the moment we met.

Deborah Sewrathan my dear friend, co-worker, and amazing oncology nurse. She once told me I should write and I took her words to heart. I appreciate her professional advice and her friendship.

Mary Govantes, exceptional oncology nurse. Her feedback and suggestions were truly appreciated.

Keri Kowalchuk, who painstakingly read through the entire manuscript, double-checking every resource. She offered sage advice in developing a format for the book. I value her input and am blessed to call her my friend.

Sharon Y. Cobb, professional screenwriter and workshop instructor at University of North Florida. Her workshops were invaluable in providing me the tools I needed to move from writer to author.

Dr. Sadir Alwari and Dr. Leonard Schvartzman, deft surgeons, skilled at their profession. Their genuine warmth and compassion made such a difference in helping me get through a difficult time my life. I could not have asked for a better cancer care team.

My patients. Their strength and courage have been an inspiration to me.

About the Author

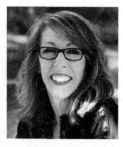

Deborah Gomer graduated from New York University with a Bachelor of Science in Nursing. She has been in practice as an oncology nurse for 25-plus years. She served as past-president of the Broward Oncology Nursing Society and was named a leader in oncology nursing by the Oncology Nursing Society. She was also honored to be named Case Manager of the Year and Health Care Super Hero by her peers. She earned certification as a case manager in 2002 and became a certified health coach in 2014. Deborah has been invited to speak to healthcare professionals and the community and has been published in various magazines for cancer survivors. She is an avid yoga practitioner and enjoys gardening and cooking. She currently resides in Florida with her family.

CPSIA information can be obtained
at www.ICGtesting.com
Printed in the USA
LVOW13s2032240518
578384LV00012B/1063/P